PATCH MANUAL

CONTENTS

MW00904215

PATCH MANUAL

LifeWave New Member Training Manual

by Dr. Jen O'Sullivan, BCND

www.jenosullivan.com www.patchedu.com

Written and designed by Jen O'Sullivan, including cover, typography, typesetting, and book design. Photography and Illustrations by various artists from Shutterstock. Cover illustration by ESB Professional.
Editors: Sandra Kozij, Karen Flinn, Kathy Schwanke, Diane Fischer, Karen Roper, Diane Finefrock, Jennifer Slan, Lisa Stockman, Regina Cocolin, Christine Perpall Rodriguez, Rene Tate, Angela Sanderson, Peggy Spurk, Jenny Chan, Nicholette Holderrieth, and Suzanne Holt.

Disclaimer: This manual is for educational purposes only. It is not intended to give medical advice or be used to diagnose, treat, cure, or prevent any disease or illness. The protocols and usage descriptions have not been evaluated by the FDA. Please check with your medical doctor prior to embarking upon any lifestyle changes.

Published by 31 Publishing, a division of 31 Oils, LLC
Published in California, USA
ISBN: 9798342055796

PATENT NO. US 10,716,953 B1

X39 is "a wearable phototherapy apparatus that produces beneficial effects to a human body such as **activation of stem cells, improvement in strength, improvement in stamina, pain relief** via a non-transdermal container. The non-transdermal apparatus reflects or emits specific wavelengths of light to **elevate levels of the copper peptide GHK-CU in the body.**"

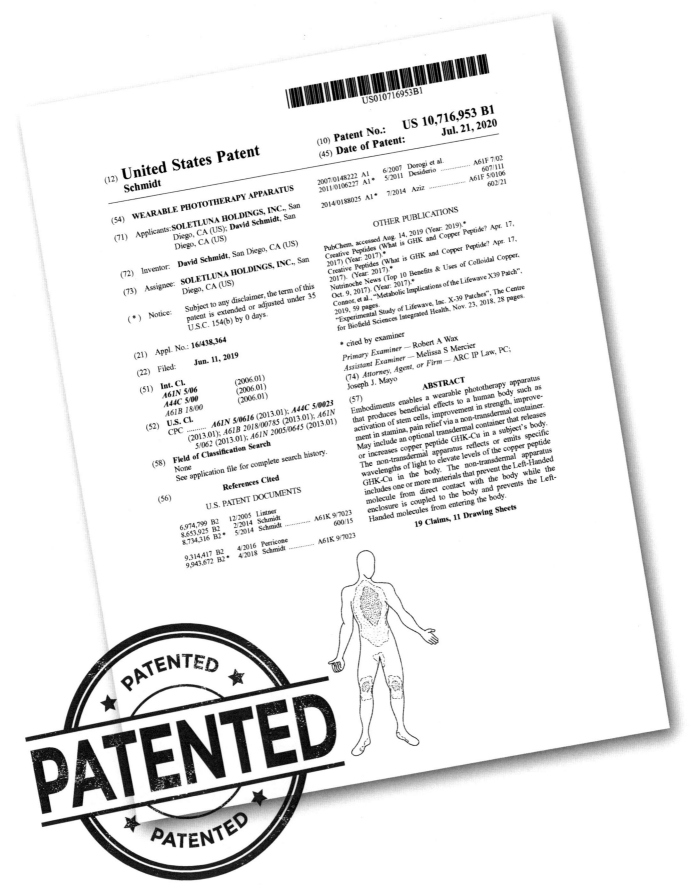

US010716953B1

(12) **United States Patent**
Schmidt

(10) Patent No.: **US 10,716,953 B1**
(45) Date of Patent: **Jul. 21, 2020**

(54) **WEARABLE PHOTOTHERAPY APPARATUS**

(71) Applicants: **SOLETLUNA HOLDINGS, INC.**, San Diego, CA (US); **David Schmidt**, San Diego, CA (US)

(72) Inventor: **David Schmidt**, San Diego, CA (US)

(73) Assignee: **SOLETLUNA HOLDINGS, INC.**, San Diego, CA (US)

(*) Notice: Subject to any disclaimer, the term of this patent is extended or adjusted under 35 U.S.C. 154(b) by 0 days.

(21) Appl. No.: **16/438,364**

(22) Filed: **Jun. 11, 2019**

(51) Int. Cl.
A61N 5/06 (2006.01)
A44C 5/00 (2006.01)
A61B 18/00 (2006.01)

(52) U.S. Cl.
CPC **A61N 5/0616** (2013.01); **A44C 5/0023** (2013.01); **A61B 2018/00785** (2013.01); **A61N 5/062** (2013.01); **A61N 2005/0645** (2013.01)

(58) Field of Classification Search
None
See application file for complete search history.

(56) **References Cited**

U.S. PATENT DOCUMENTS

6,974,799 B2	12/2005	Lintner	
8,653,925 B2	2/2014	Schmidt	A61K 9/7023
8,734,316 B2*	5/2014	Schmidt	600/15
9,314,417 B2	4/2016	Perricone	
9,943,672 B2*	4/2018	Schmidt	A61K 9/7023

2007/0148222 A1	6/2007	Dorogi et al.	A61F 7/02
2011/0106227 A1*	5/2011	Desiderio	607/111
2014/0188025 A1*	7/2014	Aziz	A61F 5/0106 602/21

OTHER PUBLICATIONS

PubChem, accessed Aug. 14, 2019 (Year: 2019).*
Creative Peptides (What is GHK and Copper Peptide? Apr. 17, 2017) (Year: 2017).*
Creative Peptides (What is GHK and Copper Peptide? Apr. 17, 2017). (Year: 2017).*
Nutrinoche News (Top 10 Benefits & Uses of Colloidal Copper, Oct. 9, 2017). (Year: 2017).*
Connor, et al., "Metabolic Implications of the Lifewave X39 Patch", 2019, 59 pages.
"Experimental Study of Lifewave, Inc. X-39 Patches", The Centre for Biofield Sciences Integrated Health, Nov. 23, 2018, 28 pages.

* cited by examiner

Primary Examiner — Robert A Wax
Assistant Examiner — Melissa S Mercier
(74) Attorney, Agent, or Firm — ARC IP Law, PC; Joseph J. Mayo

(57) **ABSTRACT**

Embodiments enables a wearable phototherapy apparatus that produces beneficial effects to a human body such as activation of stem cells, improvement in strength, improvement in stamina, pain relief via a non-transdermal container. May include an optional transdermal container that releases or increases copper peptide GHK-Cu in a subject's body. The non-transdermal apparatus reflects or emits specific wavelengths of light to elevate levels of the copper peptide GHK-Cu in the body. The non-transdermal apparatus includes one or more materials that prevent the Left-Handed molecule from direct contact with the body while the enclosure is coupled to the body and prevents the Left-Handed molecules from entering the body.

19 Claims, 11 Drawing Sheets

PATENTED ★ PATENTED ★ PATENTED

PATCH PLACEMENT GUIDE

For each patch, choose one desired location from the guide below. Try different spots each day to find which spot works best for you, or rotate daily through a few spots and observe your body's response. Wear patches for 12 hours and then remove for 12 hours before applying a new one. Some patches may be worn for 24 hours as long as you are not wearing that same patch type again for at least 24 hours. You may wear up to four different patches during any one 12-hour period. You may wear different patches during the nighttime 12-hour period. Always use X39, then complement your health regimen with several other patches.

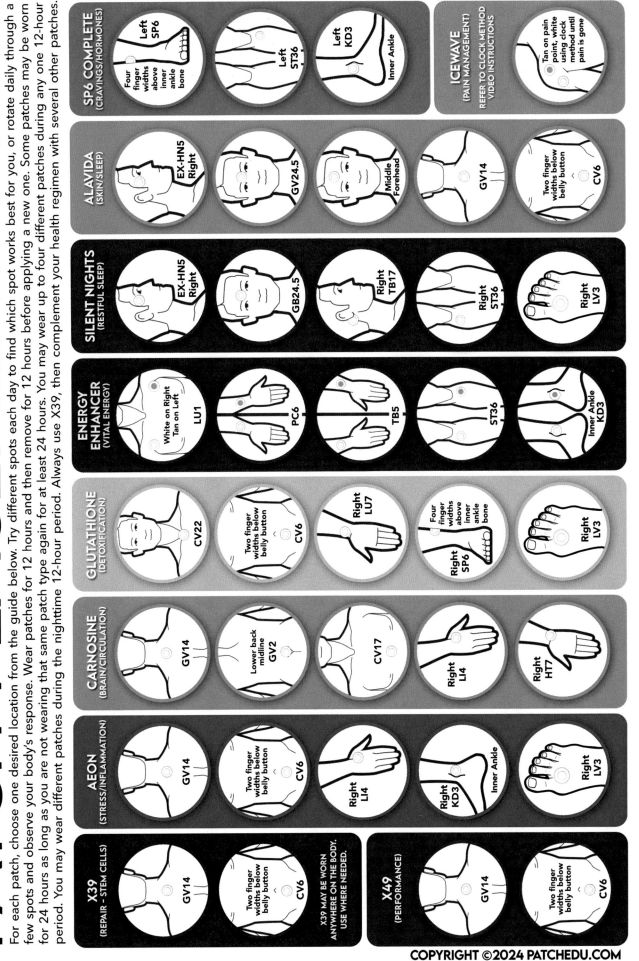

SP6 COMPLETE (CRAVINGS/HORMONES) — Left SP6, Four finger widths above inner ankle bone; Left ST36; Left KD3, Inner Ankle

ICEWAVE (PAIN MANAGEMENT) — REFER TO CLOCK METHOD VIDEO INSTRUCTIONS. Tan on pain point, white method using clock method until pain is gone

ALAVIDA (SKIN/SLEEP) — EX-HN5 Right; GV24.5; Middle Forehead; GV14; CV6, Two finger widths below belly button

SILENT NIGHTS (RESTFUL SLEEP) — EX-HN5 Right; GB24.5; Right TB17; Right ST36; Right LV3

ENERGY ENHANCER (VITAL ENERGY) — White on Right Tan on Left LU1; PC6; TB5; ST36; Inner Ankle KD3

GLUTATHIONE (DETOXIFICATION) — CV22; CV6, Two finger widths below belly button; Right LU7; Right SP6, Four finger widths above inner ankle bone; Right LV3

CARNOSINE (BRAIN/CIRCULATION) — GV14; GV2, Lower back midline; CV17; Right LI4; Right H7

AEON (STRESS/INFLAMMATION) — GV14; CV6, Two finger widths below belly button; Right LI4; Right KD3, Inner Ankle; Right LV3

X39 (REPAIR – STEM CELLS) — GV14; CV6, Two finger widths below belly button. X39 MAY BE WORN ANYWHERE ON THE BODY. USE WHERE NEEDED.

X49 (PERFORMANCE) — GV14; CV6, Two finger widths below belly button

X39 HEALTH TRACKER

The proper use of LifeWave® X39 has been proven to significantly increase GHK-Cu copper peptide in the body. Bodily production of human GHK-Cu copper peptide has been scientifically proven to increase healthy stem cell activity. Wear X39 for 12 hours per 24-hour period giving yourself a 12-hour break before applying a new X39 patch. Do this for a minimum of 6-12 months, and then continue daily use to maintain your benefits. Use this health tracker to determine your starting points and progress. Get regular doctor check-ups at the 6 and 12 month marks to track any internal or unfelt internal progress. At your check-up, ask for a basic and comprehensive metabolic panel, complete blood count, lipid panel, thyroid panel, C-reactive protein test, and vital nutrient levels. If possible, get a check-up before starting X39 (optional).

NAME: **START DATE:**

HEALTH BENEFITS – Rate yourself on a scale of 1-10 with 1 being poor health and 10 being perfect health.

	BEFORE USE	24 HOURS	WEEK ONE	WEEK TWO	MONTH ONE	MONTH TWO	MONTH THREE	MONTH FOUR	MONTH FIVE	MONTH SIX	MONTH SEVEN	MONTH EIGHT	MONTH NINE	MONTH TEN	MONTH ELEVEN	MONTH TWELVE
Mobility																
Clarity																
Energy																
Stamina																
Strength																
Recovery																
Sleep Quality																
Hormones																
Skin Health																
Nail Health																
Hair Health																
Vision Health																
Gum Health																
Moods																
Patience																
Motivation																
Other																

SYMPTOM RELIEF – Rate yourself on a scale of 1-10 with 1 being low and 10 being high.

	BEFORE USE	24 HOURS	WEEK ONE	WEEK TWO	MONTH ONE	MONTH TWO	MONTH THREE	MONTH FOUR	MONTH FIVE	MONTH SIX	MONTH SEVEN	MONTH EIGHT	MONTH NINE	MONTH TEN	MONTH ELEVEN	MONTH TWELVE
Inflammation																
Pain																
Fatigue																
Neuropathy																
Headaches																
Migraines																
Brain Fog																
Scar Tissue																
Blood Pressure																
Bad Cholesterol																
Thyroid Function																
Adrenal Function																
Other																

PATCH SCHEDULER

When you first start out using patch-based phototherapy, it is best to stick with just the X39 and Aeon patches for the first month. Adding additional patches early on may cause heavier detox symptoms. If you decide to use other LifeWave patches, it is recommended to use no more than 3-4 during each 12 hour "on" period. This means you can wear 3-4 different patches during the day such as X39, X49, Aeon, and SP6, then up to four different patches at night such as Alavida, Carnosine, and Silent Nights. Some users find they can wear 4-5 different patches per cycle, but it is important to listen to your body. If you are wearing more than four patches at one time, and you feel "off", remove one or two patches, and remember to drink a lot of water and get more electrolytes into your diet.

The patches are stabilized for a total of 24 hours, however this changes with the amount of heat the patch is subjected to, such as a hot shower, hot tub, or ambient heat above 85 degrees. Along with a brand-new patch, you can apply a used patch of the same kind the next day using medical fabric tape to any area of your body that needs extra support. You may also simply take it off after 12 hours and apply it directly to another person or even on your pet's collar. If you activate a patch, use it for 12 hours, take it off with the intentions of using it again the next day, but then forget to apply it, the patch will break down completely after around 48 hours or sooner based on initial heat exposure. Previously activated patches are dead after 36-48 hours based on how long initial use was and heat temperatures.

The X39 patch has been studied and proven to be most effective when worn in a consistent cycle of 12 hours on and 12 hours off. Wearing X39 for 24 hours on and 24 hours off will cause your progress to slow by 50%, meaning instead of seeing great results after 6 months, you may need to wait up to 12 months. Patches may be used for 24 hours if you do not plan to wear them daily. An example of this would be if you use the Y-Age trio on rotation. The Y-Age trio consists of Aeon, Carnosine, and Glutathione. Many users wear X39 daily, 12 hours on and 12 hours off, with a 24 hour rotation of the Y-Age trio.

TIMING EXAMPLE: Apply X39 and Aeon on Monday at 9am. Remove X39 at 9pm, but continue to wear Aeon until 9am the next day. Apply a new X39 on Tuesday along with Carnosine. Remove X39 at 9pm and continue to wear Carnosine until 9am the next day. On Wednesday, apply a new X39 along with Glutathione. Remove X39 at 9pm and continue to wear Glutathione until 9am the next day. Start the rotation again on Thursday with X39 and Aeon.

NAME:								START DATE:					

DATE	MONDAY		TUESDAY		WEDNESDAY		THURSDAY		FRIDAY		SATURDAY		SUNDAY	
AM DAY TIME	Time ON	Time OFF	Time ON	Time OFF	Time ON	Time OFF	Time ON	Time OFF	Time ON	Time OFF	Time ON	Time OFF	Time ON	Time OFF
X39														
X49														
Aeon														
Carnosine														
Glutathione														
Energy Enhancer														
IceWave														
SP6 Complete														
PM NIGHT TIME	Time ON	Time OFF	Time ON	Time OFF	Time ON	Time OFF	Time ON	Time OFF	Time ON	Time OFF	Time ON	Time OFF	Time ON	Time OFF
Alavida														
Silent Nights														
OPTIONAL PM														
IceWave														
Aeon														
Carnosine														
X39														

FIRST STEPS

Welcome to the LifeWave family! This Patch Manual will be your go-to resource for everything pertaining to LifeWave patches. LifeWave patches are a unique and innovative technology that combines proven science and results that empower you to obtain optimal health. Let's begin!

FIRST STEPS FOR NEW CUSTOMERS & BRAND PARTNERS
❏ Step 1: Contact your enroller for product/business questions, never customer service.
❏ Step 2: Use customer service (live chat) only for order, shipping, or account related issues.
❏ Step 3: Log into www.lifewave.com to re-order or check order status.
❏ Step 4: Who is your Sponsor (person who enrolled you)? _____
❏ Step 5: What is your member number? _____
❏ Step 6: What is your password? _____

RESOURCES
❏ Step 7: Bookmark these websites
    www.LifeWave.com
    www.LifeWaveSuccessLibrary.com
    www.YouTube.com/@PatchEDU
    www.PatchEDU.com

❏ Step 8: Get Educated
    • **PRODUCT EDUCATION**
      www.tinyurl.com/PatchEducation
    • **BUSINESS EDUCATION**
      www.tinyurl.com/BizEducation

❏ Step 9: Join the Facebook Groups
    PatchEDU LifeWave Education at www.facebook.com/groups/x39edu
    Plus, join the various groups offered by your LifeWave leadership.

❏ Step 10: Join the Weekly Online Meetings
    Join the various online meetings, classes, and events offered by your leadership.

❏ Step 11: Learn About the Patches
    X39 – Increases GHK-Cu – for rapid repair of cells and increase of healthy stem cell activity
    X49 – Increases AHK-Cu – supports performance, stamina, bone, muscle, hair, and cardiovascular
    Aeon – Reduces inflammation, helps manage stress, and supports the liver
    Alavida – For skin regeneration and smoothing, plus increases melatonin for sleep
    Carnosine – A major antioxidant for brain health to help clear brain fog and support circulation
    Energy Enhancer – Supports natural vital energy by burning fat and converting it into energy
    Glutathione – Detoxes all organs, increases glutathione by 300-400% in 24 hours
    IceWave – For specific localized pain alleviation
    Silent Nights – Supports more restful sleep at night
    SP6 Complete – Helps with food and hunger cravings, plus supports hormone balancing
    AcuLife – Designed for horses to help with pain and inflammation

These statements have not been evaluated by the FDA. These products are not intended to treat, cure, or prevent any disease.

ACCOUNT BASICS

HOW TO SIGN UP WITH LIFEWAVE
- Go to www.LifeWave.com
- Use the link or member number of the person who shared LifeWave with you
- Make sure it says at the top that you are shopping with the right person
- Click JOIN and select one of the starter packages (see the order form on page 60)
- Go through the steps to complete checkout, review your order, then hit submit
- You will see a confirmation page with your member number
- You will get several emails from LifeWave with order and subscription confirmations

HOW TO GET THE RIGHT HELP
PRODUCT QUESTIONS:
- Contact the person who enrolled you for product related questions

SHIPPING/ACCOUNT QUESTIONS:
- First option (fastest): Use Live Chat on www.LifeWave.com
- Second option: Email customerservice@lifewave.com
- Third option (not recommended due to long hold times): Call 1-866-202-0065

HOW TO REORDER MORE PATCHES
- Log into your account at www.LifeWave.com
- Always continue to upgrade through the Premium package if you did not start there
- UPGRADE: Go to "Store" at the top, then click on "Upgrade Kits"
- SUBSCRIPTION: Go to "Store" at the top, find the item, then create a subscription
- MAINTENANCE: Go to "Store" at the top, then click on "Maintenance Kits"
- ONE TIME ORDER: Go to "Store" at the top, then find an item and buy

HOW TO STAY ACTIVE & KEEP YOUR POINTS
- You only need 55PV per month to remain active
- Manager rank and above needs 110PV per month to remain active
- Remaining active keeps your points accumulating for up to a year
- Points are for cycle bonuses, not product
- Cycle Bonus eligibility: 330 on small leg (Profit Leg), 660 on big leg (Power Leg), must have one personally sponsored active Brand Partner on each leg

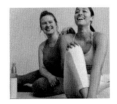
Preferred Customer Program
Get rewarded for your loyalty

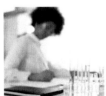
Our Product Difference
Discover our innovative health technology

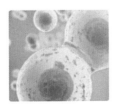
Our Story
Helping people since 2004

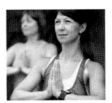
Become a Brand Partner
Become a brand partner and join our community

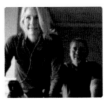
FAQs
Got Questions? We've got answers!

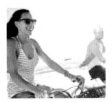
Brand Partner Stories
Discover what it means to be a brand partner

PATCH OVERVIEWS

X39 for REPAIR & LONGEVITY – increases human copper-bound tripeptide of glycine, histidine, and lysine called GHK-Cu. GHK-Cu copper peptide is known to support the proliferation and activation of healthy stem cells. GHK-Cu also has the ability to reset 4,192 genes to a younger and healthier state. Because X39 elevates GHK-Cu production in the body, it supports cellular repair, relief of inflammatory pain, wound healing, skin, hair, and nail health, hormone balancing, better energy, better sleep quality, plus it supports brain balancing to lessen depression, anxiety, aggression, and mood swings. SOURCE: tinyurl.com/X39Research

X49 for PERFORMANCE & BONE HEALTH – increases copper-bound tripeptide of alanine, histidine, and lysine which is known as AHK-Cu. AHK-Cu also decreases NTx, which is a marker for bone growth and density. Alanine supports the body's response to physical performance, strength, stamina, and recovery. X49 also supports cardiovascular health, cognitive functions, as well as increases bone density, muscle gain, and fat loss during more intense types of workouts or athletic performances. Alanine has been anecdotally studied by practitioners to increase the body's ability to withstand electromagnetic frequency (EMF) by creating a type of whole-body cellular Faraday cage when used with X39. SOURCE: tinyurl.com/X49Study

AEON for STRESS & INFLAMMATION – increases glutamate, cysteine, glutamine, serine, and proline. Aeon is considered the anti-aging patch by the inventor, David Schmidt. It helps to reduce inflammation, cortisol, C-reactive proteins, and stress. It elevates SOD (superoxide dismutase) which is important for your body's stress response, and balances the autonomic nervous system, as well as helps balance hormonal production. It is known as the "happy" patch and is likened to consuming 30 cups of Royal Jelly per day. SOURCE: tinyurl.com/AeonStudy

ALAVIDA for SKIN SMOOTHING & SLEEP – increases epithalamin and melatonin. Alavida improves the health of your skin from the inside out. Alavida elevates epithalamin, a peptide known for cellular anti-aging that helps repair chromosomes. This reduces the appearance of fine lines and wrinkles, brightens the complexion, and helps to even out skin tone and discoloration. It also helps the body to produce natural melatonin to support restful and reparative sleep. SOURCE: tinyurl.com/AlavidaStudy

CARNOSINE for BRAIN & CIRCULATION – increases beta-alanyl-L-histidine, also known as carnosine. Carnosine is a dipeptide of beta-alanine and histidine. The Carnosine patch helps your body increase the production of carnosine. Carnosine is a dipeptide found in the body that is known to improve cognitive function and help prevent mental decline and visual degeneration. It also enhances athletic performance by supporting strength, stamina, flexibility, and by lowering lactic acid production. Having more carnosine in your body has been linked to keeping your telomeres from shortening, which is important to live a long healthy life. SOURCE: tinyurl.com/CarnosineStudy

ENERGY ENHANCER for VITAL ENERGY – The Energy Enhancer patch is a two-patch system and is clinically proven to induce cellular beta-oxidation to burn fat and convert it to vital energy. It is a natural, non-transdermal nootropic that supports the increase of energy production in the cells. This patch has been clinically proven to increase overall energy and endurance naturally without the use of stimulants or drugs. It is best utilized when active. SOURCE: tinyurl.com/EnergyEnhancerStudy

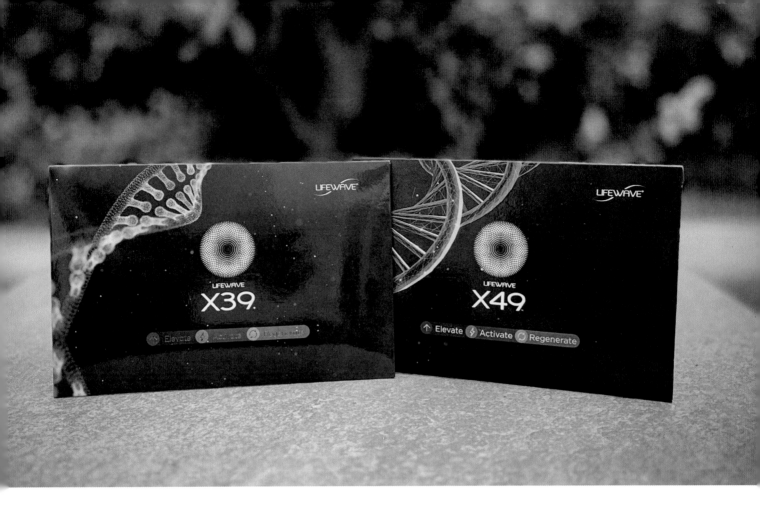

GLUTATHIONE for DETOXIFICATION – clinically proven to elevate the production of endogenous human glutathione in the body. Glutathione is the body's master antioxidant that supports organ and cellular detoxification. This patch is clinically proven to elevate glutathione levels by an average of 300-400% within 24 hours when used for one 24-hour cycle. SOURCE: tinyurl.com/GlutathioneStudy

ICEWAVE for PAIN RELIEF – increases mitochondrial activity and many amino acids. IceWave is a safe and effective solution for all levels of pain, both chronic and acute. IceWave is a two-patch system designed to help the user pinpoint and eliminate specific pain. Like all LifeWave patches, IceWave is non-transdermal, has zero drugs, is non-addictive, and has no harmful side effects. SOURCE: tinyurl.com/IceWaveStudy

SILENT NIGHTS for SLEEP – increases serotonin, which increases melatonin in low light. Silent Nights helps your body produce its own melatonin through an increase in serotonin during low light environments. It works without the use of drugs or chemicals. It is clinically proven to improve the quality and length of sleep without morning grogginess. SOURCE: tinyurl.com/SilentNightsStudy

SP6 COMPLETE for CRAVINGS & HORMONES – reduces sugar cravings and balances hormones. The SP6 Complete patch helps suppress cravings and hunger naturally by gently stimulating the SP6 acupressure point. SP6 supports any weight reduction program without the use of drugs, stimulants, or needles. It supports the health of the liver, pancreas, kidneys, thyroid, hypothalamus, adrenals, and intestines. SOURCE: tinyurl.com/SP6Study

These statements have not been evaluated by the FDA. These products are not intended to treat, cure, or prevent any disease.

FREQUENTLY ASKED QUESTIONS

HOW DO I USE THE X39 PATCH?
Place X39 at the base of your neck or two finger widths below your belly button, or anywhere on your body that you want extra support. Wear a new X39 patch each day for 12 hours and then remove and take a 12-hour break from X39. After your 12-hour break, apply a new X39 patch the next day. This is called the 12/12 method. Do this consistently every single day for a minimum of six months. You can wear it up to 16 hours per day, but make sure you give yourself at least an 8-hour break every day so as to not cause attenuation.

WHAT IS ATTENUATION?
Attenuation is when you use something too often and it becomes less effective. If you wear a LifeWave patch for 24 hours per day, seven days per week, after around 30 days of this type of use, your body will stop responding to that specific patch. The most beneficial usage for X39 is to wear 12 hours on and 12 hours off. For patches you wear for 24 hours, such as Glutathione, you may wear them 24 hours on and at least 24 hours off.

WHAT IF I FORGET AND WEAR X39 FOR 24 HOURS?
You can apply a new X39 patch and keep going or take a 12 to 24-hour break. If you consistently forget and wear X39 for 24 hours every day, give yourself a 24 to 48-hour break every five days of 24-hour use and try to get back onto a 12/12 schedule. You will see faster results with the 12/12 schedule and slower results with a 24/24 schedule.

CAN I USE THE X39 PATCH EVERY OTHER DAY AND STILL GET RESULTS?
Skipping a day of X39 will interfere with your progress. You need to stay on X39 for 6 months for the full benefits. If you wear X39 every other day it will take up to 12 months to see results.

CAN I WEAR THE X39 PATCH AT NIGHT INSTEAD OF THE DAY?
Some find it easier to wear X39 at night during the detox phase. You may continue to wear at night as needed.

WHAT HAPPENS AFTER I HAVE USED X39 FOR A FULL 6 MONTHS? CAN I STOP?
If you want to continue to experience the full benefits of X39, you will want to continue to use it. If you choose to go on a maintenance schedule you may try 24 hours on, 24 hours off. Please pay close attention to your body as you may need to continue using the 12/12 schedule.

WHAT ARE THE INGREDIENTS OF LIFEWAVE PATCHES?
They are very precisely and specifically engineered using nanoparticle crystals that are made out of organic amino acids, salts, and sugar embedded as a lattice onto polyester fabric encased by medical-grade plastic.

I AM WORRIED ABOUT USING STEM CELLS. WHERE ARE THEY COMING FROM?
There is nothing in the patches that is going into your body. They are non-transdermal. Only your own infrared body light is being reflected back. With X39, the stem cells come from your own body! The X39 triggers your body to stimulate three amino acids to combine with copper and this creates healthy active stem cells.

HOW DO DIFFERENT PATCHES CAUSE DIFFERENT RESPONSES?
This is how phototherapy works. Consider the sun. It does not have vitamin D in it. The sun hits the skin and the body produces vitamin D. In the patches, they are all different. Each crystal reflects a specific wavelength of light onto the dermis of the skin signalling your body to produce specific amino acids or biological responses. The crystals are embedded differently in each patch to elicit a specific response from the body.

DO I HAVE TO STICK THE PATCHES ON MY SKIN?
No, you can also stick the patches to the inside or outside of your clothing.

PATCH MANUAL

CAN I WEAR PATCHES IN THE SHOWER?
Yes, however if you take very hot showers, it will speed up the crystal breakdown.

CAN I WEAR PATCHES IN THE POOL?
Yes, they are waterproof. Make sure when you apply a patch, your skin is completely clean and dry.

WHAT IF A PATCH FALLS OFF DURING A WORKOUT OR FROM BEING IN WATER?
You can reapply the patch once it is dry using paper tape.

CAN I WEAR LIFEWAVE PATCHES IN AN INFRARED SAUNA OR DURING RED LIGHT THERAPY?
Yes, however if you are in a very hot environment (90s and above), it will break down the crystals faster.

WILL NICOTINE PATCHES INTERFERE WITH X39 OR VICE VERSA?
No, Lifewave patches will not interfere with nicotine patches.

CAN I GO THROUGH THE SECURITY SCANNER AT THE AIRPORT WITH MY PATCHES?
Yes, there is no issue with security scanners. The scanners will not activate your patches.

IS THERE A WAY TO ACTIVATE THE PATCHES WITHOUT KNOWING IT?
Yes, if your pet sleeps on top of the mail and your patches are in the pile, the pet will activate them all. If you carry your patches in your pocket or in a handbag close to your body and there is heat in the 80-90s, they will activate. Keep unused patches out of heat and also away from infrared human or animal light.

IS THERE A GOOD WAY TO CARRY OR TRAVEL WITH MY PATCHES?
For travel, put patches into a RFID blocking wallet or container such as a metal tin and keep out of heat.

CAN I WEAR PATCHES DURING A BODY SCAN SUCH AS AN X-RAY OR MRI?
Yes, you may wear patches during medical scans. They will not interfere.

CAN YOU WEAR TWO X39 PATCHES ON THE SAME DAY?
Yes, you may wear two X39 for extra healing. It will increase the efficacy by 20%. Do this only as needed.

CAN I STORE PATCHES IN THE CAR?
Please do not store the patches in a car where it may become too hot as they will become ineffective.

IN THE SUMMER MY HOME IS ABOVE 80 DEGREES. HOW SHOULD I STORE MY UNUSED PATCHES?
If you live in a hot area and do not keep your home cool (below 80), you will want to put your unused patch sleeves into an airtight Ziploc container and keep them in your refrigerator.

WHAT IF MY PATCHES SHIP IN THE HEAT?
Patches have stabilizers in them to keep them from activating during shipping. If your patches end up in a hot mail box for longer than a week or there is a shipping delay, contact LifeWave for a replacement.

WHAT IF MY PATCHES SHIP IN THE RAIN AND THE PACKAGE GETS WET?
As long as the inner sleeves are not wet, your patches are fine. If the inner sleeves are wet and the patch sticker backings are damaged, you may contact LifeWave for a replacement.

WHAT SHOULD I EXPECT FOR DETOX?
When you start using the patch, your body will start going to work! You may experience fatigue or other normal detox symptoms such as a headache. This is normal but can be minimized by drinking more water and getting electrolytes in your body. Take an Epsom salt bath every so often. You may start slowly by using it for six hours the first day, then use that same patch for six hours the second day. You can do this method for two to four days at which point you should start using a new patch 12 hours daily.

WHEN WILL I START NOTICING BENEFITS?
Some feel improvement in as little as minutes to even seconds, while some can take a day or a couple weeks or even months. For long-term chronic issues, it can take up to six months to see changes and in some extreme cases it can take 12 months to start noticing results. It is best to get normal labs and checkups done during your 6 months of usage (doctor, dentist, eye doctor). Some results are happening internally that you would not feel or see.

WHAT TESTS SHOULD I ASK FOR AT MY DOCTOR VISIT?
At your check-up, ask for a basic and comprehensive metabolic panel, complete blood count, lipid panel, thyroid panel, C-reactive protein test, and vital nutrient levels. If possible, get a check-up before starting X39.

WHAT IF I DO NOT SEE OR FEEL ANY BENEFITS AFTER A COUPLE MONTHS?
It may take six months to a year to see/feel benefits depending on your health condition. See above.

WHAT IF I DO NOT SEE OR FEEL ANY BENEFITS AT ALL?
There are several factors that come into play with this question: extreme health and extreme diseases. If you are very healthy, and have zero health issues, you won't notice much, but your body will heal faster when injured, and your body will age slower. They are still working. If you are very ill and/or have mineral and vitamin deficiencies, it will take a lot longer. Follow these steps: Drink 4-5 ounces of fresh water every 30 minutes. Consume proper electrolytes, namely sodium, magnesium, and potassium. If you are copper deficient, the patches need copper to bind to, so take a good quality copper supplement. Most people get enough copper in their diet, but some do not. Get blood tests done to check or take nano colloidal copper.

CAN I USE LIFEWAVE PATCHES ON PETS AND CHILDREN?
It is best to use the AcuLife patches for horses. The patches are not labeled for use on children or pets. It is up to the parent or pet owner to use at their own discretion. These are non-invasive and non-transdermal.

CAN I USE MULTIPLE PATCHES?
It is best to stick with just the X39 and Aeon for the first month. Adding additional patches early on will cause much heavier detox symptoms. If you decide to use other patches, it is recommended to use no more than 3-4 during each 12 hour "on" period. This means you can wear three different patches during the day such as X39, X49, and Aeon, then up to three different patches at night such as Alavida, Carnosine, and Silent Nights.

HOW LONG DOES EACH PATCH LAST?
The patches are stabilized for a total of 24 hours, however this changes with the amount of heat the patch is subjected to. Generally, you can expect to get 16-24 hours out of one patch. Along with a brand-new patch, you can apply used patches the next day using medical fabric tape to any area of your body you need extra support. You may also simply take it off after 12 hours and apply it directly to another person or even on your pet's collar. If you activate a patch, use it for 12 hours, take it off with the intention of using it again the next day, but then forget, the patch will break down completely after around 36 hours or sooner based on initial heat exposure. Previously activated patches are dead after 36-48 hours based on how long initial use was and temperatures.

AREN'T LIFEWAVE PATCHES LIKE OTHER PATCHES?
No, there is nothing like LifeWave patches on the market anywhere in the world. While other patches mask issues, our patches trigger peptides and amino acids to actually produce positive biological changes in the body.

IS THERE RESEARCH TO BACK UP THE INCREDIBLE CLAIMS ABOUT X39?
Yes! Please see the science section on the website www.PatchEDU.com for more information.

I LIVE IN A VERY HOT LOCATION. WILL THE PATCHES BE OK DURING SHIPPING?
Yes, LifeWave has extensively tested the stability of the patches during shipping to warm locations. If the package gets put in direct sun while you are out of town for over a week, call customer service for a replacement.

I'M ALLERGIC TO MOST ADHESIVES, CAN I USE LIFEWAVE PATCHES?
Very, very few people have a response to the adhesive. If you do, the good news is that you can wear these facing the opposite way. Simply apply the patch to the inside of your clothing or adhere with paper tape.

ARE LIFEWAVE PATCHES FSA OR HSA ELIGIBLE?
FSAs and HSAs are both ways to help you save for qualified medical expenses such as out of network treatments like chiropractic. Some FSA or HSA plans allow LifeWave patches, and some do not. Check with your provider.

CAN PREGNANT WOMEN USE THE PATCHES?

They are completely non-invasive but you should always consult your doctor. LifeWave and the brand partners of LifeWave are not allowed to give health advice to those who are pregnant.

WILL X39 INTERFERE WITH MEDICATIONS?

There are no safety precautions other than to monitor your progress if you are on any medications. As your body heals, your medications may prove to be too strong. Please work closely with your doctor to adjust your doses of medications. Basically, think of it like this: these help to reset your organs. If you're on blood pressure medications, the patches can help reset your cardiovascular system so you want to monitor yourself. If you're diabetic, you must check your blood sugar. It can help your pancreas start functioning better so you may end up really drowsy and nauseous if you don't monitor your blood closely.

WILL THE X39 DETOX MY MEDICATIONS?

The X39 will NOT detox any medications or treatments. If this were the case, then ALL medications would be detoxed too quickly when using X39. This is not the case.

IS X39 SAFE DURING CHEMOTHERAPY?

X39 gives your body a 30% increase in glutathione levels. Many doctors want patients who are undergoing chemotherapy

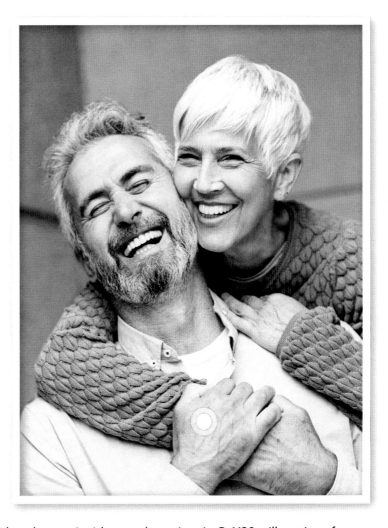

to limit or not use any supplement that is considered an antioxidant such as vitamin C. X39 will not interfere with your treatment, but each person is welcome to decide for themselves what is right for them. Some choose to wear the patch the day after treatment, and up to the day before, and not use X39 the day of. LifeWave and the brand partners of LifeWave are not allowed to give health advice to cancer patients.

I AM AN ORGAN TRANSPLANT PATIENT. IS X39 SAFE FOR ME TO USE?

X39 gives your body a 30% increase in glutathione levels. Many patients with a donor organ use X39 without issue. LifeWave and the brand partners of LifeWave are not allowed to give health advice to those with specific issues. It is up to you as a transplant recipient to choose your personal health practices.

IS THERE ANYONE THAT CANNOT USE LIFEWAVE PATCHES?

Technically no, everyone can use them. From a legal standpoint, no one is allowed to give treatment advice to anyone including pregnant women, cancer patients, and organ transplant patients. Doing so is considered practicing medicine without a license. It is illegal for anyone except a medical doctor to give diagnostic or treatment advice for any disease or illness to others. It puts you and the company at risk. It is up to them if they want to use this non-invasive phototherapy product.

ABOUT LIFEWAVE

LIFEWAVE COMPANY STATISTICS

- Founded in 2004 by inventor, owner, and CEO David Schmidt
- Open in over 70 countries worldwide
- Innovative and patented products that no one else provides
- X39 pre-launched in late 2018 with the official launch in 2019
- X39 took $4.5 million and 10 years to develop
- Growth rate of 3,000% from 2018-2024
- LifeWave went from a $20 million company to over $600 million per year in five years
- The fastest growing network marketing company in the world
- Winner of the 2024 Direct Selling News (DSN) Bravo Growth Award
- Ninth largest network marketing company in the world based on growth rate

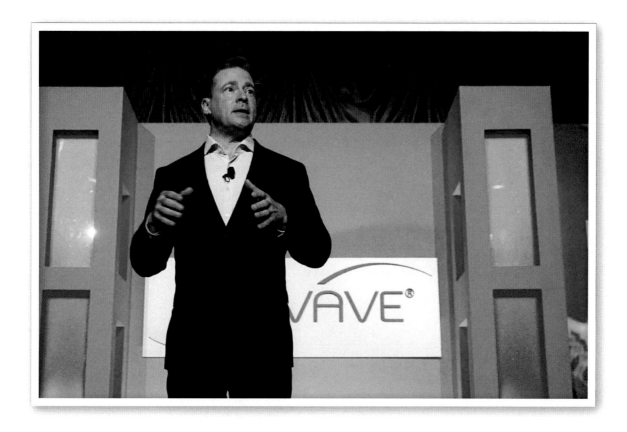

ABOUT DAVID SCHMIDT

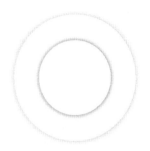

DAVID SCHMIDT
- Scientist, inventor, founder, and CEO of LifeWave
- David holds over 150 patents
- LifeWave has over 80 clinical trials on their patches
- David is an Honorary Doctor of Science and Technology
- David is a two-time recipient of the Advanced Technology Award from the International Hall of Fame

FROM "THE STORY OF X39" BY DAVID SCHMIDT

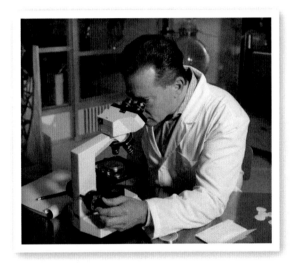

"Independent third-party clinical studies on GHK-Cu have determined some remarkable benefits including, support of the body's natural wound healing process. Perhaps even more remarkably, GHK-Cu resets the genes in the body to a younger, healthier state. In initial clinical work performed by Dr. Loren Pickart, Dr. Pickart discovered that old liver cells, when exposed to GHK-Cu, started to function like younger, healthier cells!"

"I founded LifeWave in 2002 as a research company based on a new technology that I had invented (and later patented) for improving health with a new form of phototherapy. In August of 2004, we went to market and LifeWave was an immediate success, generating $17 million in sales in our very first year. Since then, LifeWave has become a global company with offices in the United States, Ireland, and Taiwan, and distribution to more than 100 countries. LifeWave has truly become an international success story."

DAVID'S TYPICAL DAILY PATCHING ROUTINE
- X39 behind the neck on the GV14 acupoint
- X49 below the navel at the CV6 acupoint
- Energy Enhancer on the upper chest at the LU1 acupoints
- Aeon on right upper shin muscle at the ST36 acupoint or various points as needed
- Alavida on the right temple at the EX-HN5 acupoint at bedtime

ACUPRESSURE

Acupressure is part of the Traditional Chinese Medicine (TCM) modality of healing that stimulates the flow of energy to promote well-being. It is based on the same principles as acupuncture, but instead of using needles, acupressure relies on manual pressure on specific body points called acupoints. LifeWave patches use pressure by stimulating the skin with infrared light from your body. Acupressure also involves working with the body's meridian system. This system is a network of energy channels through which vital life force, or Qi, flows. By applying stimulation with LifeWave patches to specific acupoints along meridians, energy flow blockages can be released, promoting balance and healing.

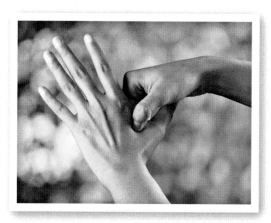

COMMON ACUPOINT LOCATIONS

*There are over 400 acupoints. This list only covers some of the popular locations for patching. Each acupoint lists main benefiting body systems or symptoms, but not all. Acupoints with an * are the most commonly used points in patch therapy.*

BL23 (Bladder 23) "Shenshu" – Kidney/Urine regulation
At the second lumbar spinal nerve on lower back

CV4 (Conception Vessel 4) "Guan Yuan" – Digestion
A hand width below navel

*CV6 (Conception Vessel 6) "Qi Hai" – Qi/Hormones
Two finger widths below navel

CV12 (Conception Vessel 12) "Zhong Wan" – Digestion
Six finger widths above the navel

CV17 (Conception Vessel 17) "Dan Zhong" – Heart/Cough
Breastbone in line with nipple

CV22 (Conception Vessel 22) "Tian Tu" – Sore Throat/Cough
The hollow at the base of the throat

*EX-HN5 "Taiyang" – Headaches/Eye/Sinus
Temple on side of face

GV2 (Governing Vessel 2) "Yao Shu" – Back Pain
Lowest midline back point

*GV14 (Governing Vessel 14) "Dazhui" – Brain/Inflammation
Back of neck at the C7 vertebra

GV24.5 (Governing Vessel 24.5) "Yin Tang" – Headache/Stress
Between eyebrows (third eye)

HT7 (Heart 7) "Shenmen" – Anxiety/Addiction/Migraine
Inner wrist in line with the pinky finger

*K1 (Kidney 1) "Yongquan" – Headache/Fever/Dizziness
Just behind ball of foot

K3 (Kidney 3) "Tai Xi" – Fertility/Tinnitus/Low Back Pain
Between inner ankle bone and Achilles tendon

*LI4 (Large Intestine 4) "Hegu" – Skin/Dark Circles
Hand muscle between thumb and pointer finger

LI5 (Large Intestine 5) "Yangxi" – Head/Eye Swelling
Wrist crease in line with thumb

LI20 (Large Intestine 20) "Ying Xiang" – Cold/Sinus
On cheeks next to nostrils

LU1 (Lung 1) "Zhong Fu" – Cough/Asthma/Wheezing
Outside upper chest just above underarm

LU7 (Lung 7) "Lie Que" – Flu/Cold/Fever
Below inner wrist crease in line with thumb

*LV3 (Liver 3) "Taichong" – Blood Pressure/Irritability
Top of foot between big toe and second toe

*PC6 (Pericardium 6) "Neiguan" – Nausea/Insomnia
Two finger widths from inner wrist crease

*SP6 (Spleen 6) "Sanyinjiao" – Cravings/Vertigo/Sleep
Four finger widths above inner ankle bone

ST25 (Stomach 25) "Tian Shu" – Diarrhea/Constipation
Two finger widths to the side of the navel

*ST36 (Stomach 36) "Zusanli" – Digestion/Leg Strength
Top of shin muscle when flexing foot up

TB5 (Triple Burner 5) "Wai Guan" – Immune/Allergies
Two finger widths from outer wrist crease

TB17 (Triple Burner 17) "Yifeng" – Ear Issues/Vertigo
Behind earlobe on neck

These statements have not been evaluated by the FDA. This guide is not intended to treat, cure, or prevent any disease.

ACUPOINT LOCATIONS

For patch placement using LifeWave patches, please refer to the specific patches and recommended locations on the inside cover, and also in the Protocols section starting on page 32.

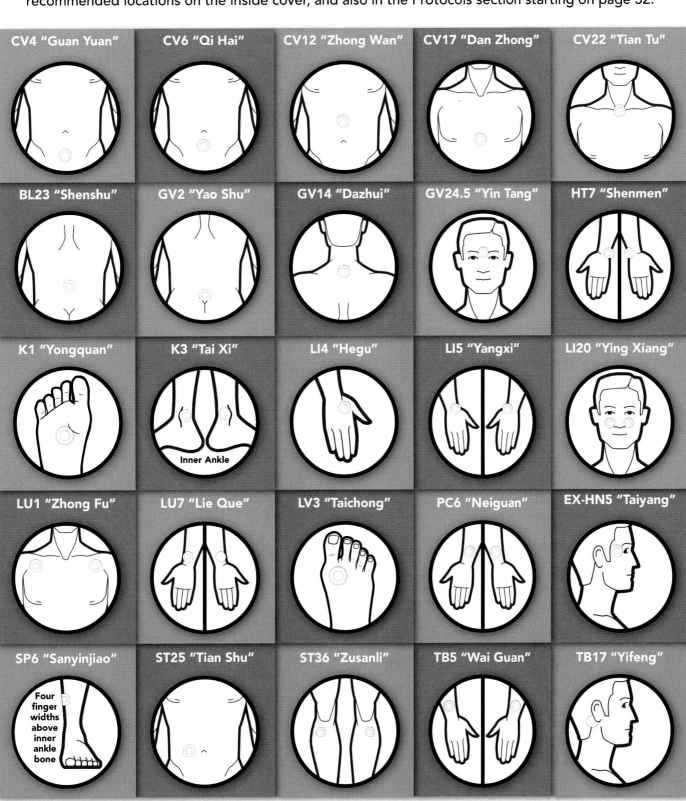

CV4 "Guan Yuan" CV6 "Qi Hai" CV12 "Zhong Wan" CV17 "Dan Zhong" CV22 "Tian Tu"

BL23 "Shenshu" GV2 "Yao Shu" GV14 "Dazhui" GV24.5 "Yin Tang" HT7 "Shenmen"

K1 "Yongquan" K3 "Tai Xi" LI4 "Hegu" LI5 "Yangxi" LI20 "Ying Xiang"

Inner Ankle

LU1 "Zhong Fu" LU7 "Lie Que" LV3 "Taichong" PC6 "Neiguan" EX-HN5 "Taiyang"

SP6 "Sanyinjiao" ST25 "Tian Shu" ST36 "Zusanli" TB5 "Wai Guan" TB17 "Yifeng"

Four finger widths above inner ankle bone

AMINO ACIDS & PEPTIDES

Amino acids are crucial to the proper function of various biological processes. They are essential for the structure and function of cells, tissues, and organs in the body, which is why they are often referred to as the building blocks of proteins. Peptides are made up of a string of amino acids; anywhere from two to 50 different amino acids can make up a peptide. A dipeptide is when two amino acids join together. A tripeptide is when three join. Polypeptides are longer strings of more amino acids joined together.

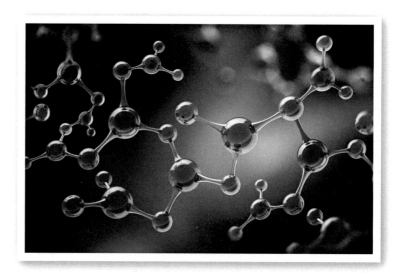

AMINO ACID BENEFITS & FUNCTIONS
There are 20 amino acids, nine of which are essential.

ESSENTIAL – Your body doesn't produce

HISTIDINE (X39, X49, Carnosine*, IceWave*)
Supports growth, tissue repair, makes blood cells, and protects nerve cells. It is used to make histamine. Histamine supports immune function, digestion, and improved sleep.
Deficiency Diseases: Anemia, slow wound healing, poor cognition and memory, arthritis

ISOLEUCINE (Energy Enhancer*)
Supports immune function, muscle metabolism, energy production, and hemoglobin production.
Deficiency Diseases: Hypoglycemia, dizziness, mental decline, depression, fatigue, weight loss

LEUCINE (X49, SP6 Complete*)
Supports athletic muscle recovery, improves strength and stamina, heals wounds, regulates blood sugar, and balances hormones.
Deficiency Diseases: Lethargy, weight loss, skin rashes, hair loss

LYSINE (X39, X49, Energy Enhancer*)
Supports calcium absorption, collagen production, hormone production, energy, and immune system health, and helps block cortisol.
Deficiency Diseases: Fatigue, saggy skin, bone loss, agitation, anemia, nausea, loss of appetite, fatty-acid absorption issues

METHIONINE (Glutathione*)
Supports detoxification, liver health, immune health, metabolism, and mineral absorption.
Deficiency Diseases: Liver disease, kidney disease, metabolic disorder, psychosis, fatigue

PHENYLALANINE (Carnosine*)
Supports brain signaling, memory, learning, mental alertness, and more balanced moods.
Deficiency Diseases: Intellectual disability, behavioral issues, seizures

THREONINE (Alavida*)
Critical for metabolism, immune health, emotional balance, and cognition. Supports collagen, elastin, and blood clotting.
Deficiency Diseases: Multiple sclerosis, ALS, anorexia, weak immune system, fatty liver disease

TRYPTOPHAN (Alavida*, Silent Nights*, IceWave*)
Supports serotonin and melatonin production, and regulates appetite, moods, and energy.
Deficiency Diseases: Hartnup disease, pellagra, pain sensitivity, aggression

VALINE (Energy Enhancer*)
Supports energy production, muscle growth, tissue repair, focus, coordination, and emotions.
Deficiency Diseases: Insomnia, cognitive decline, loss of muscle mass, fatigue, weakness

18

NONESSENTIAL AMINO ACIDS – Your body produces these

ALANINE (X49, Carnosine*)
Creates energy for muscles, brain, and central nervous system, strengthens immune system, and supports stamina by removing lactic acid. Promotes the growth of hair and nails.
Deficiency Diseases: Loss of muscle mass, fatigue, loss of endurance and strength

ARGININE (IceWave*)
Lowers blood pressure, stimulates insulin, supports immune health, improves heart and cardiovascular health, and supports blood sugar.
Deficiency Diseases: Seizures, developmental delays, spasticity in legs, erectile dysfunction

ASPARAGINE (Aeon)
Detoxifies cellular ammonia and supports brain signals. Supports athletic performance and muscle strength, along with healthy cell growth.
Deficiency Diseases: Cognitive decline, cerebral atrophy, seizures, weak muscle tone

ASPARTIC ACID (Alavida*)
Supports energy production and supports the nervous system. Supports athletic performance, stamina, and immune system health.
Deficiency Diseases: Neural and brain disorders

CYSTEINE (Aeon, Glutathione*)
Powerful antioxidant (natural NAC). Increases collagen and keratin for hair, skin, and nails.
Deficiency Diseases: Cardiovascular, stroke, diabetes, lung/colon cancers, renal, vitiligo

GLUTAMATE (Aeon, Glutathione*)
Supports memory, cognition, learning, mood, increases GABA, and promotes sleep.
Deficiency Diseases: Autism, ADD, ADHD

GLUTAMINE (X39, Aeon)
Building block for muscles, removes toxins (ammonia), supports immune system, brain, digestion, intestines, liver, and kidney health.
Deficiency Diseases: Frequent illnesses, constipation, or diarrhea, and obesity

GLYCINE (X39, Glutathione*)
Supports muscle building, joint repair, and collagen building. Reduces inflammation, protects the liver and heart, improves metabolism and digestion, and supports improved sleep quality. Glycine is vital in Glutathione production for detoxification.
Deficiency Diseases: Fatigue, breathing issues, weak muscle tone, seizures

PROLINE (Aeon, SP6 Complete*)
Supports metabolism, skin healing, collagen, joints, cartilage, immune function, metal chelation, and reduces oxidative stress.
Deficiency Diseases: Various skin diseases, OCD, anxiety, and panic attacks

SERINE (Aeon, IceWave*)
Supports brain function, stress reduction, and immune function.
Deficiency Diseases: Parkinson, fibromyalgia, cancer, diabetes, schizophrenia, seizures

TYROSINE (X39, Aeon)
Important in synthesizing Norepinephrine (X39) and L-DOPA (Aeon). Supports melanin which is the pigment for hair/skin color. Supports adrenal, thyroid, and pituitary health.
Deficiency Diseases: Parkinson's, dystonia, cerebral palsy, abnormal gait

INCREASED AMINO ACIDS BY VARIOUS LIFEWAVE PATCHES

X39 – GHK-Cu copper-bound tripeptide of Glycine, Histidine, and Lysine
X39 also triggers Tyrosine and Glutamine
X49 – AHK-Cu copper-bound tripeptide of Alanine, Histidine, and Lysine
Aeon – Cysteine, Glutamate, Glutamine, Proline, Serine, and Tyrosine
Alavida* – Alanine, Glutamate, Aspartic Acid, Glycine, and Threonine
Carnosine* – Histidine, Alanine, and Phenylalanine
Glutathione* – Cysteine, Glutamate, Glycine, and Methionine

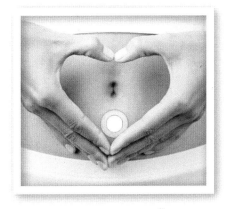

Energy Enhancer, IceWave, Silent Nights, and SP6 Complete studies do not have any information on specific amino acid improvement.

* Based on typical amino acid profiles that are utilized for this type of patch. This amino acid is not listed in any specific study for this particular patch.

These statements have not been evaluated by the FDA and are not intended to diagnose, treat, cure, or prevent any disease.

EFFECTS OF AGING

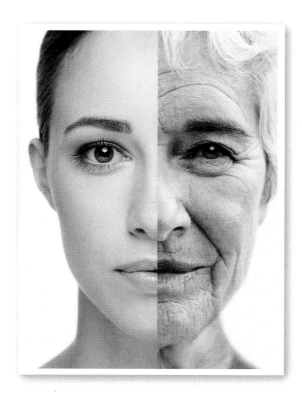

As you age, your stem cells mutate and go dormant causing wrinkles, gray hair, body aches, and organ challenges. Many factors affect why mutations happen such as our genetic makeup, environmental factors, stress, lack of sleep, poor nutrition, and so on. Unhealthy stem cells circulating in our body is one of the main reasons we experience aging, discomfort, and disease. Healthy stem cell activity drastically declines with age.

Stem cells are special cells in your body that start out as a clean slate. They are what's called undifferentiated cells, meaning they can become anything. They can become any cell in your body such as heart cells, lung cells, skin cells, blood cells, or any other type of cell that is needed. Stem cells are a main part of how our body repairs itself. Having an abundance of healthy stem cells is key to aging well.

STEM CELL DETERIORATION
- **At age 20, we have a billion healthy stem cells**
- **By age 30, healthy stem cells decline by 60% to 400 million**
- **By age 50, healthy stem cells decline by 75% to 250 million**
- **By age 60, healthy stem cells decline by 90% to 100 million**
- **By age 80, healthy stem cells decline by 95% to 50 million**

INVASIVE STEM CELL THERAPY

Invasive stem cell therapy is not FDA approved or regulated. Doctors are treating patients at the risk of losing their license, practice, and even jail-time. Interestingly, stem cell therapy has only a 30% proliferation (reproduction) rate in one localized spot and that is if it even works. In order to have a higher efficacy rate, it is always recommended that people get at least three rounds of injections. Stem cell therapy costs $5,000 to $25,000 per treatment, with three sessions needed, and zero guarantee that the patient will obtain the desired results.

GHK-CU COPPER PEPTIDE

GHK-Cu is a copper peptide that occurs naturally in your body and affects 4,192 genes. It is responsible for many critical functions in your body. It is known to help repair and reset your body in many ways. One of the most important jobs of GHK-Cu is to increase healthy stem cell activity in your body. GHK-Cu in the body declines at the same rate as stem cells, so by age 30, GHK-Cu declines by 60% and by age 60, it declines by 90%!

There are currently no GHK-Cu products on the market that are able to supplement your body the way it does on its own. Many people are turning to invasive stem cell therapy, but this has its own issues that can make this type of treatment inaccessible to the general population as well as potentially very dangerous, not to mention illegal.

GHK-Cu has been studied and proven to support optimal health in many ways. In his research, Dr. Loren Pickart has proven the relationship between elevated GHK-Cu levels and our ability to heal and stay young through healthy stem cell regeneration.

BENEFITS OF GHK-CU COPPER PEPTIDE

- Activates healthy stem cells
- Reduces inflammatory response
- Supports cardiovascular health
- Supports neurological health
- Supports nerve regeneration
- Improves collagen production
- Improves skin and nail strength
- Increases hair growth/thickness
- Improves lung tissue repair
- Reduces anxiety and aggression
- Helps improve strength/stamina
- Supports reduced recovery time
- Improves memory/mental clarity
- Supports more restful sleep
- Promotes healthy stress response
- Supports balanced emotions
- Improves hormone balance
- Improves wound healing
- Induces scar tissue remodeling
- Supports free radical absorption

When the body produces GHK-Cu copper peptide, mitochondria are involved in regulating the balance between the amount and quality of GHK-Cu that is produced. Mitochondria provide the necessary energy and metabolic support for GHK-Cu proliferation (growth and increase). GHK-Cu stimulates blood vessel and nerve outgrowth (regeneration), increases collagen, elastin, as well as supports the function of dermal fibroblasts, which are the main cell type present in skin connective tissue (dermis).

SOURCES/STUDIES
tinyurl.com/GHK-Cu
tinyurl.com/LorenPickart

PHOTOTHERAPY

LifeWave patches use patented organic nanocrystal technology and work through photobiomodulation (a type of phototherapy) and acupressure. When applied, it reflects specific wavelengths of infrared light from your body at specific acupoints, which then signals your body to work toward optimal energy flow. A good example of how phototherapy works is with the sun. When sunlight hits your skin, your body is signaled to create vitamin D. With LifeWave patches, your body's own infrared light is being reflected back to trigger the production of various amino acids and peptides depending on the patch used.

GHK-CU AND MITOCHONDRIA
In the case of X39, it produces a copper peptide called GHK-Cu. As the dermis of the skin is stimulated by X39, mitochondria are activated, causing the body to produce more GHK-Cu. Mitochondria are involved in regulating the balance between the amount and quality of GHK-Cu that is produced. Mitochondria provide the necessary energy and metabolic support for GHK-Cu proliferation (growth and increase).

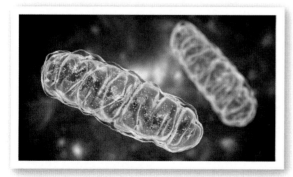

Mitochondria play a crucial role in our bodies. They are responsible for generating most of the energy needed to power various cellular processes through a process called cellular respiration. This is where mitochondria produce adenosine triphosphate (ATP), which serves as the energy currency of every cell.

When your body is properly hydrated, drinking four to five ounces of water every 30 minutes, along with getting the right electrolytes, mitochondria thrive and can greatly impact your body's ability to produce GHK-Cu.

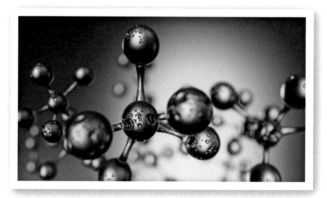

GHK-CU COPPER PEPTIDE
GHK-Cu copper peptide has been studied and proven to support optimal health in many ways. In his research, Dr. Loren Pickart has proven the relationship between elevated GHK-Cu levels and our ability to heal and stay young. Essentially, GHK-Cu has astounding cell-protective and regenerative properties. A 2018 study published in the International Journal of Molecular Sciences by Dr. Loren Pickart and Anna Margolina states,

"The human peptide GHK (glycyl-l-histidyl-l-lysine) has multiple biological actions... It stimulates blood vessel and nerve outgrowth, increases collagen, elastin, and glycosaminoglycan synthesis, as well as supports the function of dermal fibroblasts. GHK's ability to improve tissue repair has been demonstrated for skin, lung connective tissue, boney tissue, liver, and stomach lining. GHK has also been found to possess powerful cell protective actions, such as multiple anti-cancer activities and anti-inflammatory actions, lung protection and restoration of chronic obstructive pulmonary disease (COPD) fibroblasts... anti-anxiety, anti-pain, and anti-aggression activities, DNA repair, and activation of cell cleansing via the proteasome system."

THE X39 SOLUTION

HOW X39 WORKS

The X39 patch by LifeWave® elevates GHK-Cu copper peptide in your body that will, in turn, activate your stem cells to proliferate like they did in your 20s, without all the mutations. X39 activates the mitochondrial energy centers of your cells, which then increases healthy stem cell activity by resetting 4,192 genes back to how they originally performed!

The X39 patch works by using a form of phototherapy, called photobiomodulation, that uses patented non-invasive, nanocrystal technology. Our bodies emit a form of infrared light that activates the patch causing it to reflect very specific wavelengths of light that stimulate the skin. This triggers your body to produce different peptides and amino acids that then cause biochemical changes in the body. The X39 patch triggers GHK-Cu copper peptide.

THE SOLUTION

The X39 patch is patented technology that is clinically proven to significantly increase GHK-Cu copper peptide concentrations in the body along with healthy, youthful stem cells. X39 is a safe, effective, and affordable way to reset 4,192 genes back to when you were young.

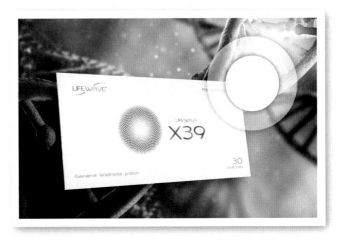

X39 FACTS

- Proven to activate healthy stem cells
- Proven to increase GHK-Cu copper peptide
- Patented and clinically proven technology
- Patent No. 10,716,953 B1
- Ingredients: amino acids, salt, and/or sugar
- FDA recognized "General Wellness Product"
- Class 1 Medical Device
- Non-transdermal and non-invasive
- Waterproof and shower-proof
- High-density medical-grade plastic
- Medical-grade hypoallergenic adhesive
- 96% effective and very affordable!

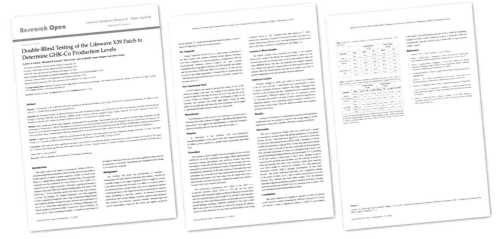

DOUBLE-BLIND TEST

A double-blind test published in the "Internal Medicine Research - Open Journal" showed a significant increase in copper-peptide concentrations in the blood of subjects who had worn the X39 patches for only one week.

STUDY:
tinyurl.com/X39research

These statements have not been evaluated by the FDA. This product is not intended to treat, cure, or prevent any disease.

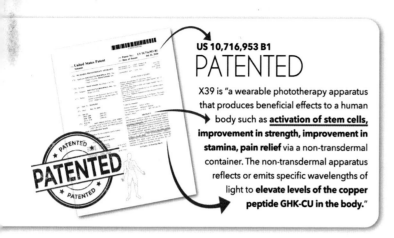

US 10,716,953 B1
PATENTED

X39 is "a wearable phototherapy apparatus that produces beneficial effects to a human body such as **activation of stem cells, improvement in strength, improvement in stamina, pain relief** via a non-transdermal container. The non-transdermal apparatus reflects or emits specific wavelengths of light to **elevate levels of the copper peptide GHK-CU in the body.**"

PATENTED TECHNOLOGY

X39 Patent Number: US 10,716,953 B1
X39 is "a wearable phototherapy apparatus that produces beneficial effects to a human body such as activation of stem cells, improvement in strength, improvement in stamina, and pain relief via a non-transdermal container. The non-transdermal apparatus reflects or emits specific wavelengths of light to elevate levels of the copper peptide GHK-Cu in the body."

ABOUT X39

- Proven to activate healthy stem cells
- Proven to increase GHK-Cu copper peptide
- Uses phototherapy to trigger healing
- Patented and clinically proven technology
- Made out of amino acids, salt, and/or sugar
- FDA recognized "General Wellness Product"
- Class 1 Medical Device
- Non-transdermal and non-invasive
- Contains no drugs or stimulants
- Waterproof and shower-proof
- High-density medical-grade plastic
- Medical-grade hypoallergenic adhesive
- 96% effective and very affordable!

HOW X39 WORKS

The X39 patch uses patented organic nanocrystal technology that works through photobiomodulation (a type of phototherapy) and acupressure. When applied to the skin, it reflects specific wavelengths of infrared light from your body back onto the skin. This signals your body to produce specific peptides and amino acids.

GHK-CU COPPER PEPTIDE

A double-blind test published in the "Internal Medicine Research - Open Journal" showed a significant increase in GHK-Cu copper peptide concentrations in the blood of subjects who had worn the X39 patches for one week.
View the study: tinyurl.com/X39research

GHK-Cu copper peptide has been studied and proven to support optimal health in many ways. In his research, Dr. Loren Pickart has proven the relationship between elevated GHK-Cu levels and our ability to heal and stay young through healthy stem cell regeneration.

**View the study: tinyurl.com/GHK-Cu
More studies: tinyurl.com/LorenPickart**

BENEFITS OF GHK-CU COPPER PEPTIDE

- Activates healthy stem cells
- Reduces inflammatory response
- Supports cardiovascular health
- Supports neurological health
- Supports nerve regeneration
- Improves collagen production
- Improves skin and nail strength
- Increases hair growth/thickness
- Improves lung tissue repair
- Reduces anxiety and aggression
- Helps improve strength/stamina
- Supports reduced recovery time
- Improves memory/mental clarity
- Supports more restful sleep
- Promotes healthy stress response
- Supports balanced emotions
- Improves hormone balance
- Improves wound healing/scars
- Supports free radical absorption

Research Source: tinyurl.com/GHK-Cu

STEM CELL DETERIORATION
At 20 we have a billion healthy stem cells
By 30 they decline by 60% to 400 million
By 50 they decline by 75% to 250 million
By 60 they decline by 90% to 100 million
By 80 they decline by 95% to 50 million

LIFEWAVE X39®

WHAT TO EXPECT WITH X39

Day One – A feeling of clarity and energy is experienced as ATP is activated and healthy stem cells begin to regenerate and increase. SCIENCE: Mitochondrial activity increases.

One Week – Clinical studies prove that after one week there is a significant increase in GHK-Cu copper peptide in the blood. SCIENCE: GHK-Cu copper peptide along with eight amino acids increase in the body.

Six Weeks – Clarity of mind with an overall sense of well-being are felt. The body goes to work where it is most needed and restoration is underway all over the body. SCIENCE: Calmer brain and moods.

Three Months – Improved performance, strength, and stamina along with reduced recovery time may be noticed. Skin may be smoother and wounds heal faster.

Six Months – Many benefits are seen at the six-month mark such as an improved stress response, balanced emotions, more clarity, deeper restful sleep, and improved hair. SCIENCE: Improved medical lab numbers.

Continued Use – Continued use gives greater benefits toward your optimal health.

STAY HEALTHY WITH X39!
The X39 patch by LifeWave is the only patented technology available in the world that is clinically proven to increase healthy stem cells in the body. With a 96% efficacy rate, backed by gold-standard research and patents, your health is in good hands with LifeWave. Stay healthy with X39 today!

X39® is an FDA recognized and compliant "General Wellness Product" and is not intended to diagnose, treat, cure, or prevent any disease or illness.

HOW TO USE X39

Wear one LifeWave X39 patch per day on the back of your neck at the GV14 acupoint or below your navel at the CV6 acupoint. You may also wear X39 anywhere on your body that needs extra

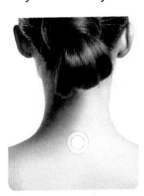

support. Use for 12 hours and then remove and discard the patch to allow your body to rejuvenate for 12 hours before using a new X39 patch the next day. X39 works wherever your body needs it most by increasing higher levels of reparative energy through healthy stem cell activation. Wear daily for at least one month per decade of life or 6-12 months for best results. Continued use will give greater benefits.

MAXIMIZE YOUR BENEFITS

- Drink 4-5 oz. of water every 30 min.
- Consume proper electrolytes daily
- Lessen processed sugar intake
- Lessen processed foods
- Eat more healthful foods
- Sweat-induced exercise daily
- Get 10-20 minutes of sunshine daily
- Take a plant-based Multivitamin
- Take CoQ10 or PQQ in the morning
- Take Turmeric before bed

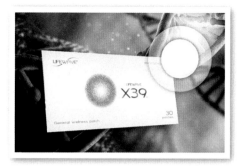

X39
THE STEM CELL PATCH

Clinically proven to increase human GHK-Cu copper peptide, which supports these benefits:

- 2100% stem cell proliferation rate
- Activates stem cells systemically
- Reduces inflammation
- Reduces stiff joints and pain
- Improves muscle and bone density
- Helps improve strength/stamina
- Supports reduced recovery time
- Increases collagen and elastin
- Increases hair growth and thickness
- Improves nail strength and health
- Eases anxiety and aggression
- Supports cardiovascular health
- Supports neurological health

- Supports nerve regeneration
- Improves lung tissue repair
- Improves memory/mental clarity
- Supports more restful sleep
- Promotes healthy stress response
- Supports balanced emotions
- Improves hormone balance
- Improves wound healing
- Supports scar tissue remodeling
- Supports free-radical absorption
- Increases Glycine for inflammation
- Increases Histidine for repair
- Increases Lysine for collagen

"A double-blind test published in the "Internal Medicine Research - Open Journal" showed a significant increase in copper-peptide concentrations in the blood of subjects who had worn the X39 patches for one week."

SOURCE: tinyurl.com/X39Research

PRO ADVICE:

- Start with X39 and Aeon daily if you have high stress and/or inflammation.
- Start with X39 and X49 daily to gain muscle and bone density or support hair growth.
- Start with X39 and SP6 daily to work on hormone balancing and weight reduction.

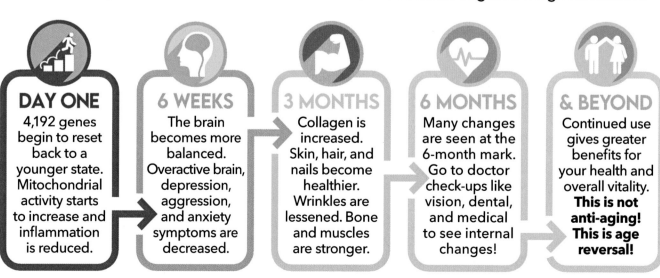

DAY ONE 4,192 genes begin to reset back to a younger state. Mitochondrial activity starts to increase and inflammation is reduced.

6 WEEKS The brain becomes more balanced. Overactive brain, depression, aggression, and anxiety symptoms are decreased.

3 MONTHS Collagen is increased. Skin, hair, and nails become healthier. Wrinkles are lessened. Bone and muscles are stronger.

6 MONTHS Many changes are seen at the 6-month mark. Go to doctor check-ups like vision, dental, and medical to see internal changes!

& BEYOND Continued use gives greater benefits for your health and overall vitality. **This is not anti-aging! This is age reversal!**

These statements have not been evaluated by the FDA. This product is not intended to treat, cure, or prevent any disease.

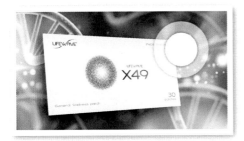

X49
THE PERFORMANCE PATCH

Clinically proven to increase AHK-Cu copper peptide, which supports these benefits:

- Increases AHK-Cu (performance)
- Decreases NTx (bone health)
- Improves strength, stamina and recovery
- Improves lean muscle mass
- Decreases bone breakdown
- Increases bone density
- Triggers dopamine and serotonin
- Enhances motivation and moods
- Supports blood vessel linings
- Supports cardiovascular health
- Supports hair and nail growth
- Reduces exposure to EMF
- Increases Alanine for performance
- Increases Histidine for repair
- Increases Lysine for collagen

"There was a significant change in both AHK-Cu and NTx. A decrease in NTx levels has been shown to correlate to a decrease in osteoclast activity, and thus a decrease in bone breakdown which means there is less bone for the osteoblastic bone formation to replace." "X49 triggered support of the dopamine pathway." "X49 triggered support for 5HT in the catecholamine pathway supporting serotonin production."

SOURCE: tinyurl.com/X49Study

These statements have not been evaluated by the FDA. This product is not intended to treat, cure, or prevent any disease.

PRO ADVICE:

- X49 works best when you use it while exercising.

- Wear X49 during a deep tissue massage.

- Wear X49 and X39 together for EMF protection.

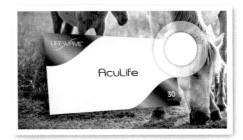

ACULIFE
THE HORSE PATCH

Clinically proven to support sensitivity and pain in horses, which supports these benefits:

- Fast-acting for immediate pain relief
- Supports improved mobility
- Reduces inflammation
- Allows for healthier engagement
- Reduces overall stress
- No drugs and non-invasive

"The overall data demonstrated that in every case there was a change in the sensitivity of the palpated points after application of the AcuLife Patches to painful points. In each case the sensitivity and pain observed were considerably lower compared to pre-patch application. The infrared thermal imaging data showed related changes as noted in palpation data sheets. In some cases, there was not just a cooling effect, but sometimes there was a warming effect: an obvious attempt of the body to balance the system. (This was quite exciting to the researchers and was indicative of the efficacy of the AcuLife Patches. In the Veterinarian's expert opinion, this is a dramatic effect. It should be noted that as we learned from our previous study last year with the horse Munoso, who's very cold area warmed, as, at the same time, the inflamed areas cooled.) "

SOURCE: tinyurl.com/AcuLifeStudy

These statements have not been evaluated by the FDA. This product is not intended to treat, cure, or prevent any disease.

PRO ADVICE:

- Directly beside the poll, on each side of the halter, place the tan patch on the left side and the white patch on the right side.

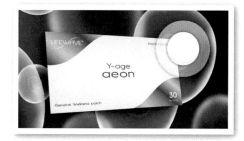

AEON
THE HAPPY PATCH

Clinically proven to improve cellular organ function and the autonomic nervous system.

- Reduces inflammation
- Supports stress response
- Supports liver function
- Reduces adrenal fatigue
- Reduces strain and tension
- Supports cognition and memory
- Enhances precursor to dopamine
- Enhances positive moods
- Supports balanced emotions
- Supports heavy metal chelation
- Supports free-radical absorption
- Increases Glutamate for GABA
- Increases Cysteine for keratin
- Increases L-DOPA for motivation
- Increases Serine for stress reduction
- Increases Glutamine for immune health
- Increases Proline for calming

"Wearing the Aeon Patch for 20 min reduces stress... (and) elicited an enhanced parasympathetic response and could enable the majority of the participants to achieve a reduced stress state with varying degrees."

SOURCES:
tinyurl.com/AeonStudy
tinyurl.com/AeonStudy2

These statements have not been evaluated by the FDA. This product is not intended to treat, cure, or prevent any disease.

PRO ADVICE:

- Start with X39 and Aeon daily if you have high stress and/or inflammation.
- May be rotated daily using the Y-Age trio of Aeon, Carnosine, and Glutathione.

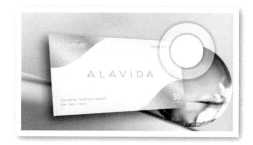

ALAVIDA
THE BEAUTY SLEEP PATCH

Elevates the production of epithalamin, which supports these benefits:

- Regulates melatonin production
- Regulates circadian rhythm
- Induces telomere elongation
- Supports chromosome repair
- Restores radiant appearance
- Reduces fine lines and wrinkles
- Promotes firmer looking skin
- Improves even skin tone and color
- Brightens the complexion
- Improves frontal lobe function
- Supports adrenal function
- Improves thyroid function
- Supports homeostasis
- Improves liver function
- Improves kidney function
- Improves pancreas function
- Supports metabolism

"Wearing a new Alavida patch... produced highly significant improvements in the physiologic functional status of the frontal lobes, hypothalamus, adrenals, thyroid gland, pituitary gland, and liver... There was a very significant improvement... in the functional status of kidneys and pancreas."

SOURCE: tinyurl.com/AlavidaStudy

These statements have not been evaluated by the FDA. This product is not intended to treat, cure, or prevent any disease.

PRO ADVICE:

- Use Alavida only at night (sleep inducing).
- Best patch location is on the right temple.
- Wear 5 nights in a row with 2 nights off.

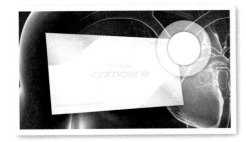

CARNOSINE
THE CLARITY PATCH

Elevates the production of carnosine in the body, which supports these benefits:

- Supports improved circulation
- Increases focus and alertness
- Improves cognitive function
- Supports healthy motivation
- Improves flexibility and balance
- Improves strength and endurance
- Lowers athletic lactic acid build-up
- Supports healthy muscle contractions
- Prevents bloodstream oxidation
- Improves liver and pancreas function
- Supports adrenal function
- Improves thyroid function
- Supports homeostasis
- Reduces cardiac stress
- Increases Alanine for performance
- Increases Histidine for repair

"The carnosine patch worn 12 hours daily on alternate days... produced a very significant improvement in the physiologic functional status of the pancreas, liver, right kidney, left and right adrenals, hypothalamus, pituitary and thyroid glands."

SOURCES:
tinyurl.com/CarnosineStudy
tinyurl.com/CarnosineStudy2

These statements have not been evaluated by the FDA. This product is not intended to treat, cure, or prevent any disease.

PRO ADVICE:

- If age 60 or above, wear Carnosine daily.

- May be rotated daily using the Y-Age trio of Aeon, Carnosine, and Glutathione.

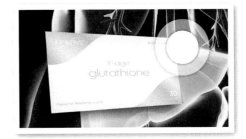

GLUTATHIONE
THE DETOX PATCH

Clinically proven to elevate the production of endogenous human glutathione in the body, which supports these benefits:

- Supports overall organ cleansing
- Supports liver and kidney detox
- Decreases acne comedones
- Supports daily stress response
- Protects mitochondria
- Supports energy production
- Increases skin elasticity
- Supports heart health
- Reduces inflammation
- Relieves spectrum symptoms
- Increases vitamin D absorption
- Supports proper methylation
- Improves immune defenses
- Increases Cysteine for redox
- Increases Glutamate for detox
- Increases Glycine for inflammation

The Glutathione causes "the body to produce more endemic glutathione. Clinical studies utilizing blood analyses indicate an average rise of more than triple (300%) the blood glutathione over a period of 24 hours." [SIC]

SOURCES:
tinyurl.com/GlutathioneStudy
tinyurl.com/GlutathioneAcne

These statements have not been evaluated by the FDA. This product is not intended to treat, cure, or prevent any disease.

PRO ADVICE:

- When new to patches, and using X39, wait one month before using Glutathione.

- May be rotated daily using the Y-Age trio of Aeon, Carnosine, and Glutathione.

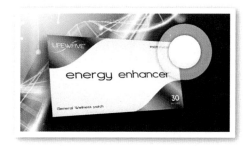

ENERGY ENHANCER

THE ENERGY PATCH

Clinically proven to induce beta-oxidation to burn fat and convert it to vital energy.

- Induces beta-oxidation
- Metabolizes and burns fat for energy
- Increases ATP (cellular energy)
- Engages natural energy field
- Improves clarity and motivation
- Supports physical activity
- Balances cognitive vitality
- Increases vital energy
- Supports metabolic function
- Supports homeostasis
- Unblocks negative energy

"Application of the LifeWave Energy Enhancer patch produced a significant increase in maximum aerobic ATP, maximum ATP from fatty acid metabolism, resting ATP, and maximum aerobic work."

SOURCE: tinyurl.com/EnergyEnhancerStudy

These statements have not been evaluated by the FDA. This product is not intended to treat, cure, or prevent any disease.

PRO ADVICE:

- Energy Enhancer patches are a two-patch system. Each package contains 30 patches (15 white and 15 tan) for a total of 15 uses.

- Wear for 12 hours on and 12 hours off for 14 consecutive days for best results.

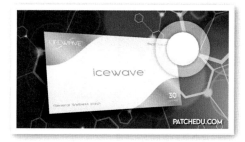

ICEWAVE

THE PAIN PATCH

Clinically proven to increase mitochondrial function and reduce pain and inflammation.

- Fast-acting for immediate relief
- Supports improved mobility
- Reduces inflammatory response
- Eases tension headaches
- Eases local acute pain
- Eases all-over body pain
- Works on chronic and acute pain
- Eases muscle tension pain
- Balances cognitive vitality
- Safe and non-addictive
- No drugs or harmful side effects

"The use of the IceWave class I medical devices for pain control have a very important and almost immediate effect on the moderation of the muscular contractions and tensions, as well as of the associated pain."

SOURCE: tinyurl.com/IceWaveStudy

These statements have not been evaluated by the FDA. This product is not intended to treat, cure, or prevent any disease.

PRO ADVICE:

- IceWave patches are a two-patch system. Each package contains 30 patches (15 white and 15 tan) for a total of 15 uses.

- May be worn for 24 hours at a time. Take 1-2 days off every 5 full days of use.

- Instructions: tinyurl.com/IceWave-Manual

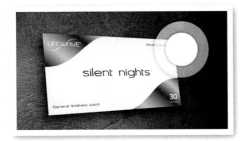

SILENT NIGHTS
THE SLEEP PATCH

Clinically proven to increase serotonin levels to promote melatonin in low light.

- Increases serotonin levels
- Induces melatonin in low light
- Supports restful sleep
- Cultivates restorative sleep
- Improves deeper sleep quality
- Increases sleep duration
- Non-habit forming
- No drugs or depressants
- Wake up refreshed
- Wake up without grogginess
- Allows for a more energized day

Wearing the Silent Nights patch, "the active group improved sleep by 2.22 hours after the 2nd week compared to baseline whereas the placebo group improved sleep by 0.98 hours in the same period."

SOURCE: tinyurl.com/SilentNightsStudy

These statements have not been evaluated by the FDA. This product is not intended to treat, cure, or prevent any disease.

PRO ADVICE:

- If starting with X39, start Silent Nights 1-2 months after you begin using phototherapy.

- Silent Nights may take several nights of usage to determine the best location. Try several locations over the course of a week to find the best spot for you.

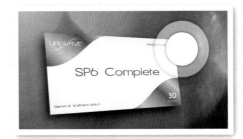

SP6 COMPLETE
THE CRAVINGS PATCH

Clinically proven to reduce cravings and improve overall hormone function.

- Supports appetite regulation
- Reduces sugar cravings
- Helps ease addiction
- Improves hormone balance
- Supports motivation
- Improves liver function
- Improves pancreas function
- Balances thyroid function
- Improves intestine function
- Supports adrenal function
- Supports kidney function
- Improves diet regimens

"The SP6 Patch worn on the ST36 acupressure point... produced a highly significant improvement in the physiologic functional status of the liver, pancreas, kidneys... the thyroid, intestines and hypothalamus... (and) the adrenal glands."

SOURCE: tinyurl.com/SP6Study

These statements have not been evaluated by the FDA. This product is not intended to treat, cure, or prevent any disease.

PRO ADVICE:

- Wear SP6 on the LEFT side of the body.

- SP6 Complete is best used on the left SP6 acupoint or the left ST36 acupoint.

30 PATCH PROTOCOLS

Each protocol lists multiple patches. Use all patches noted for best results.

ADDICTION

- SP6 Complete on left inner wrist in line with thumb (LI5)
- Aeon on right inner wrist in line with thumb (LI5)

  This can help with any type of addiction.

SUGAR ADDICTION

- SP6 Complete four finger widths above left inner ankle (SP6)

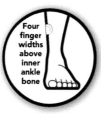

Four finger widths above inner ankle bone

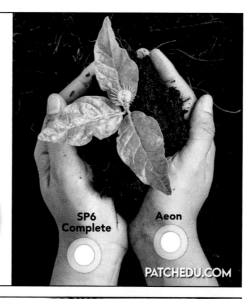

SP6 Complete   Aeon

PATCHEDU.COM

BACK PAIN

- X39 on the back of the neck (GV14)
- IceWave - tan on pain, then choose one location for white until pain is 80% improved: north, east, south, or west

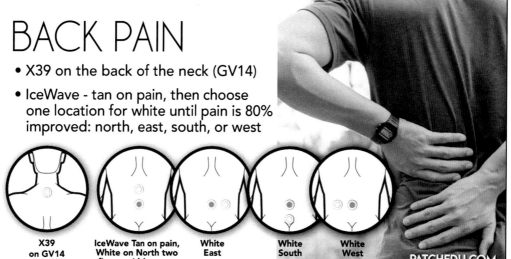

| X39 on GV14 | IceWave Tan on pain, White on North two finger widths away | White East | White South | White West |

PATCHEDU.COM

BLOATING

- Aeon on top of right hand between thumb and pointer (LI4)
- Carnosine six finger widths above the navel (CV12)

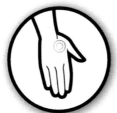
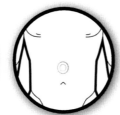

Aeon on Right LI4   Carnosine on CV12

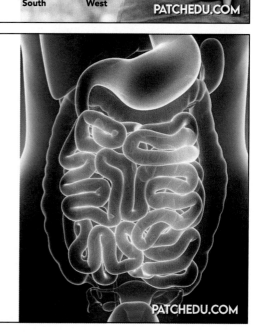

PATCHEDU.COM

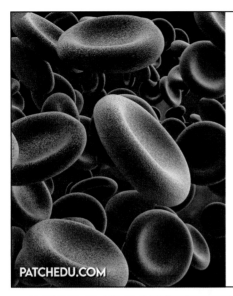

BLOOD SUGAR

- X39 on back of neck (GV14) or two finger widths below navel (CV6)
- Aeon on top of right foot (LV3)
- SP6 Complete four finger widths above left inner ankle (SP6)

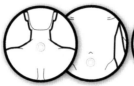
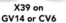
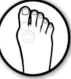

X39 on GV14 or CV6   **Aeon on right LV3**   **SP6 Complete on left SP6**

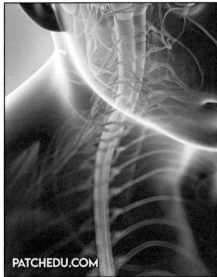

BONE HEALTH

- X39 on the back of the neck (GV14)
- X49 two finger widths below navel (CV6)

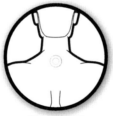
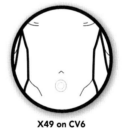

X39 on GV14   **X49 on CV6**

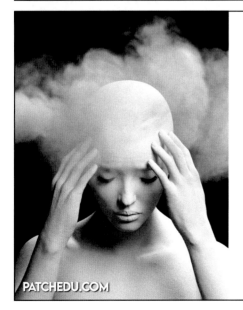

BRAIN FOG

- X39 on back of neck (GV14)
- Carnosine behind right earlobe (TB17)
- Aeon two finger widths below navel (CV6)

X39 on GV14   **Carnosine on TB17**   **Aeon on CV6**

33

CALM & FOCUS

- X39 two finger widths below navel (CV6)
- Aeon behind right earlobe (TB17)
- Carnosine/Glutathione every other day on back of neck (GV14)

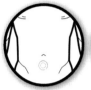

X39 on
CV6

Aeon on
TB17

Rotate Carnosine and
Glutathione on GV14

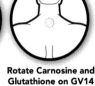

PATCHEDU.COM

CONSTIPATION TUMMY RESET PROTOCOL

Follow this rotation for 15-18 days, 12 hours on, 12 hours off.

- Day 1: Aeon six finger widths above navel (CV12), Glutathione three finger widths to the right and three finger widths above navel, SP6 Complete three finger widths to the left and three finger widths above the navel

- Day 2: Aeon one thumb width above navel, Glutathione three finger widths to the right of the navel, SP6 Complete three finger widths to the left of the navel

- Day 3: Aeon two finger widths below navel, Glutathione three finger widths to the right of the navel and three finger widths below navel, SP6 Complete three finger widths to the left of the navel and three finger widths below the navel

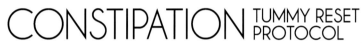
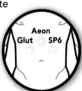

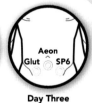

Day One   Day Two   Day Three

PATCHEDU.COM

COUGH

- Aeon at the base of sternum (CV17)
- Glutathione at the hollow at the base of the throat (CV22)

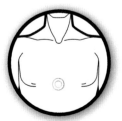

Aeon on CV17

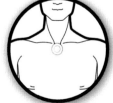

Glutathione on CV22

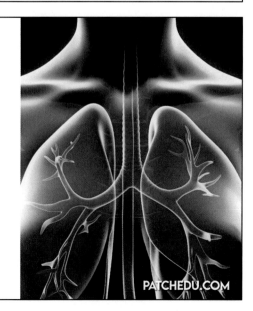

PATCHEDU.COM

34

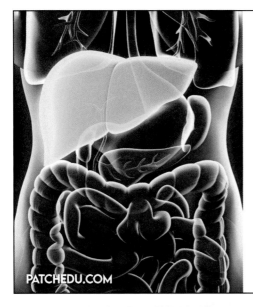

DETOX

- X39 on the back of the neck (GV14) or two finger widths below navel (CV6)
- Glutathione on right inner ankle (SP6) Wear for 24 hours every other day

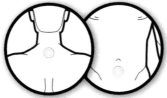
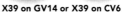
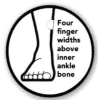

X39 on GV14 or X39 on CV6

Four finger widths above inner ankle bone

Glutathione on right SP6 point

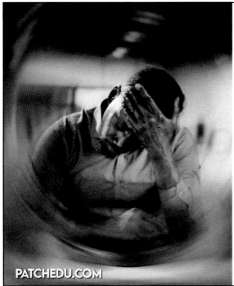

DIZZINESS

- Energy Enhancer on top of foot between big toe and second toe (LV3) White patch on right foot, tan on left

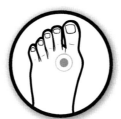
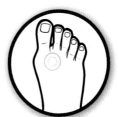

Energy Enhancer Tan on left LV3

Energy Enhancer White on right LV3

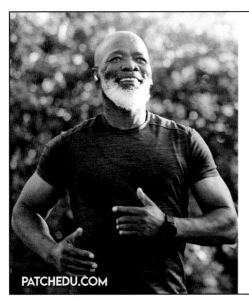

DOPAMINE RESET

- X39 on back of neck (GV14)
- X49 two finger widths below navel (CV6)
- Aeon behind right earlobe (TB17)

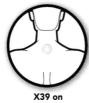

X39 on GV14

X49 on CV6

Aeon on TB17

35

EMF SHIELD

- X39 on the back of the neck (GV14)
- X49 two finger widths below navel (CV6)

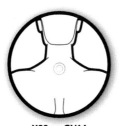

X39 on GV14

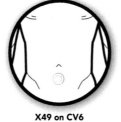

X49 on CV6

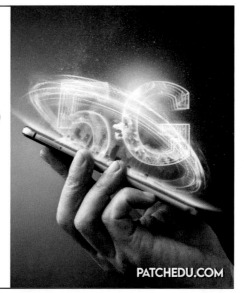

PATCHEDU.COM

EYE HEALTH

- X39 on the back of the neck (GV14)
- Carnosine on right temple (EX-HN5)

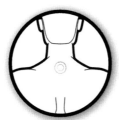

X39 on GV14

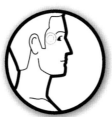

Carnosine on right EX-HN5

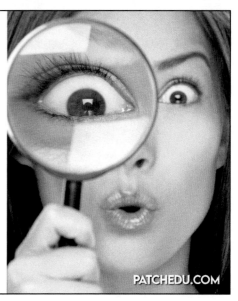

PATCHEDU.COM

HAIR HEALTH

- X39 on the back of the neck (GV14)
- X49 two finger widths below navel (CV6)

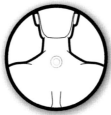

X39 on GV14

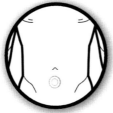

X49 on CV6

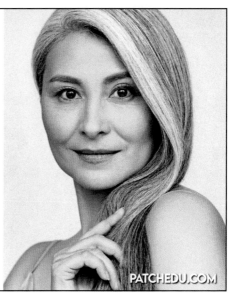

PATCHEDU.COM

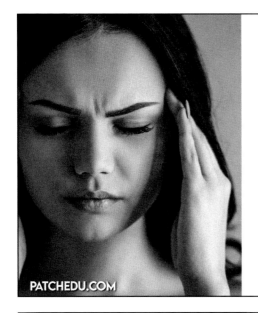

HEAD TENSION

- IceWave on temples (EX-HN5)
  White patch on right temple, tan on left

- Aeon behind right earlobe (TB17)

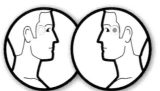

IceWave
White on right
EX-HN5

IceWave
Tan on left
EX-HN5

Aeon on
TB17

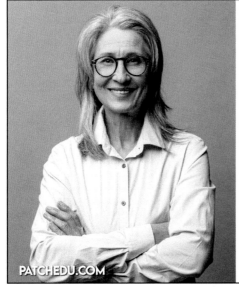

HORMONES

- X39 two finger widths below navel (CV6)
- Aeon on the back of the neck (GV14)
- SP6 Complete four finger widths
  above left inner ankle (SP6)
  or outer left shin muscle (ST36)

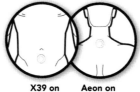
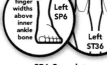

X39 on
CV6

Aeon on
GV14

Four finger widths above inner ankle bone

Left SP6

Left ST36

SP6 Complete on
left SP6 or ST36

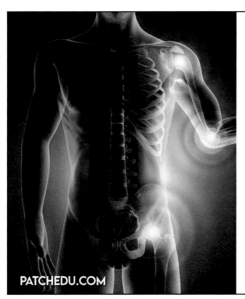

INFLAMMATION

- X39 on the back of the neck (GV14)
- Aeon two finger widths below navel (CV6)

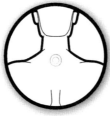
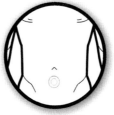

X39 on GV14

Aeon on CV6

MUSCLE BUILDING

- X39 on the back of the neck (GV14)
- X49 two finger widths below navel (CV6)

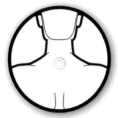

X39 on GV14

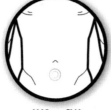

X49 on CV6

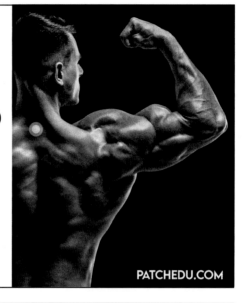

PATCHEDU.COM

NAIL STRENGTH

- X39 on the back of the neck (GV14)
- X49 two finger widths below navel (CV6)

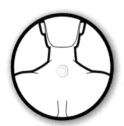

X39 on GV14

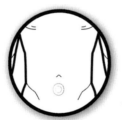

X49 on CV6

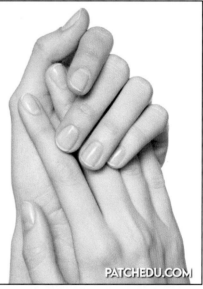

PATCHEDU.COM

PAIN CONTROL

- X39 on the back of the neck (GV14)
- IceWave on bottom of feet (K1)
  White patch on right foot, tan on left

**X39
on GV14**

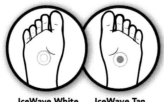

**IceWave White
on right K1**　　**IceWave Tan
on left K1**

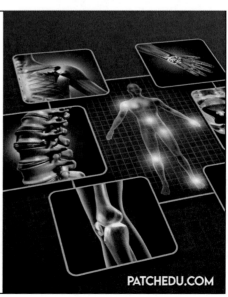

PATCHEDU.COM

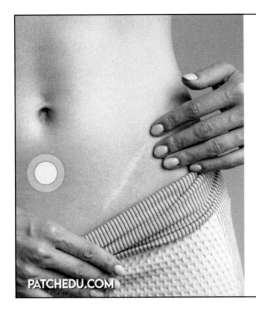

SCAR SMOOTHING

- X39 on the back of the neck (GV14)
- X49 two finger widths below navel (CV6)

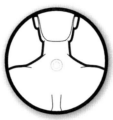
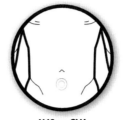

X39 on GV14 **X49 on CV6**

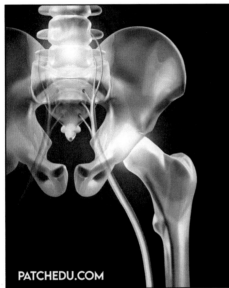

SCIATICA

- X39 on lower middle back (GV2) or the hip side where the pain is
- X39 on pain side bottom of foot (K1)

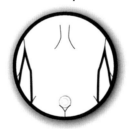
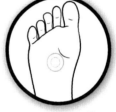

X39 on GV2 **X39 on K1 (pain side)**

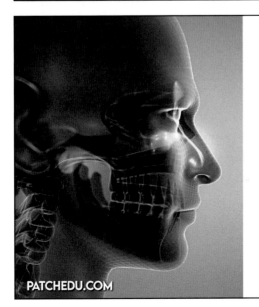

SINUS PRESSURE

- Aeon between eyebrows (GV24.5)
- Aeon on right and left cheeks next to nostrils (LI20)

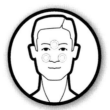

Aeon on GV24.5 and on right and left LI20

SKIN SMOOTHING

- X39 on the back of the neck (GV14)
- X49 two finger widths below navel (CV6)
- Alavida at night on right temple (EX-HN5)

X39 on GV14   X49 on CV6   Alavida on right temple at night EX-HN5

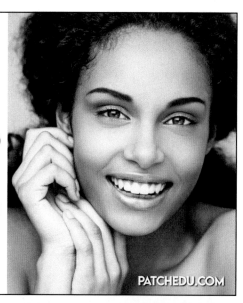

PATCHEDU.COM

SLEEP SUPPORT

- Silent Nights on side of neck behind right earlobe (TB17)
- Alavida on right temple (EX-HN5)

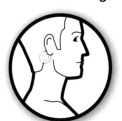 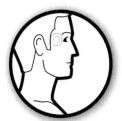

Silent Nights on right TB17   Alavida on right EX-HN5

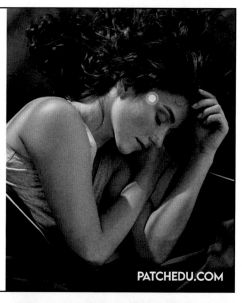

PATCHEDU.COM

SORE THROAT

- Glutathione on center of throat
- IceWave on sides of neck
  White patch on right side, tan on left
- Aeon behind right earlobe (TB17)

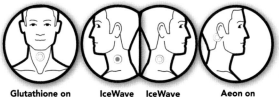

Glutathione on center of throat   IceWave tan on left side   IceWave white on right side   Aeon on TB17

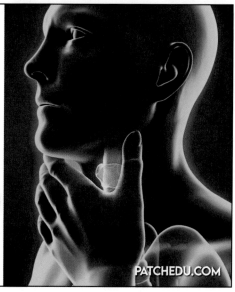

PATCHEDU.COM

40

STRESS & ANXIETY

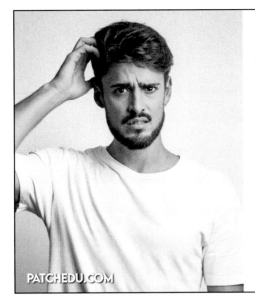

- X39 on the back of the neck (GV14)
- Aeon two finger widths below navel (CV6)

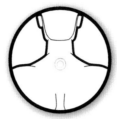
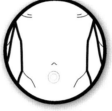

X39 on GV14 **Aeon on CV6**

PATCHEDU.COM

TINNITUS

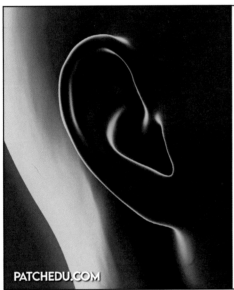

- X39 on the back of the neck (GV14)
- Energy Enhancer between inner ankle bone and Achilles tendon (K3)
  White patch on right side, tan on left

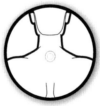
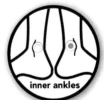

inner ankles

X39 on GV14 **Energy Enhancer on K3 (WRTL)**

PATCHEDU.COM

WEIGHT LOSS

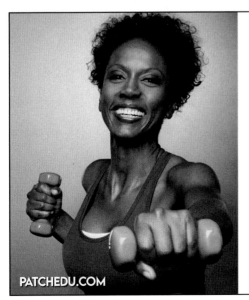

- X39 on the back of the neck (GV14) or two finger widths below navel (CV6)
- Glutathione on right inner ankle (SP6)
- SP6 Complete on left inner ankle (SP6)

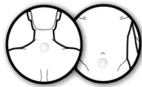

inner ankles

X39 on GV14 or CV6 **Glutathione on right inner SP6** **SP6 Complete on left inner SP6**

PATCHEDU.COM

41

LIFEWAVE 2023
INCOME DISCLOSURE STATEMENT

RANK	Percent of active Brand Partners	2023 Annual Earnings for Active Brand Partners			Average Months to Achieve Rank*
		HIGH	LOW	AVERAGE	
BRAND PARTNER	93%	$30,329	$3	**$40**	-
MANAGER	6%	$74,490	$5	**$1,709**	4
DIRECTOR	1%	$111,703	$15	**$8,217**	8
SENIOR DIRECTOR	<1%	$67,267**	$50	**$16,248**	10
EXECUTIVE DIRECTOR	<1%	$121,430	$500	**$45,677**	15
PRESIDENTIAL DIRECTOR	<1%	$203,896	$14,309	**$79,806**	16
SENIOR PRES. DIRECTOR	<1%	$2M+	$2,286	**$396,580**	24

* Measured from the date of enrollment.   ** The number for Senior Director in the "HIGH" category is correct as it is based on the highest individual payout for that rank in 2023. High means the highest any one person in that rank category was paid, low means the lowest any one person in that rank category was paid, and average is what the total average paid for all people in that rank.

The average time it takes to get to Senior Presidential Director is only two years of full time work! **What would you do with an extra $396,580 per year?**

$396,580

$79,806

$45,677

$16,248

$8,217

$1,709

$40

BRAND PARTNER · MANAGER · DIRECTOR · SENIOR DIRECTOR · EXECUTIVE DIRECTOR · PRESIDENTIAL DIRECTOR · SENIOR PRESIDENTIAL DIRECTOR

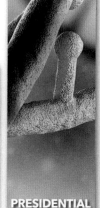

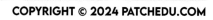

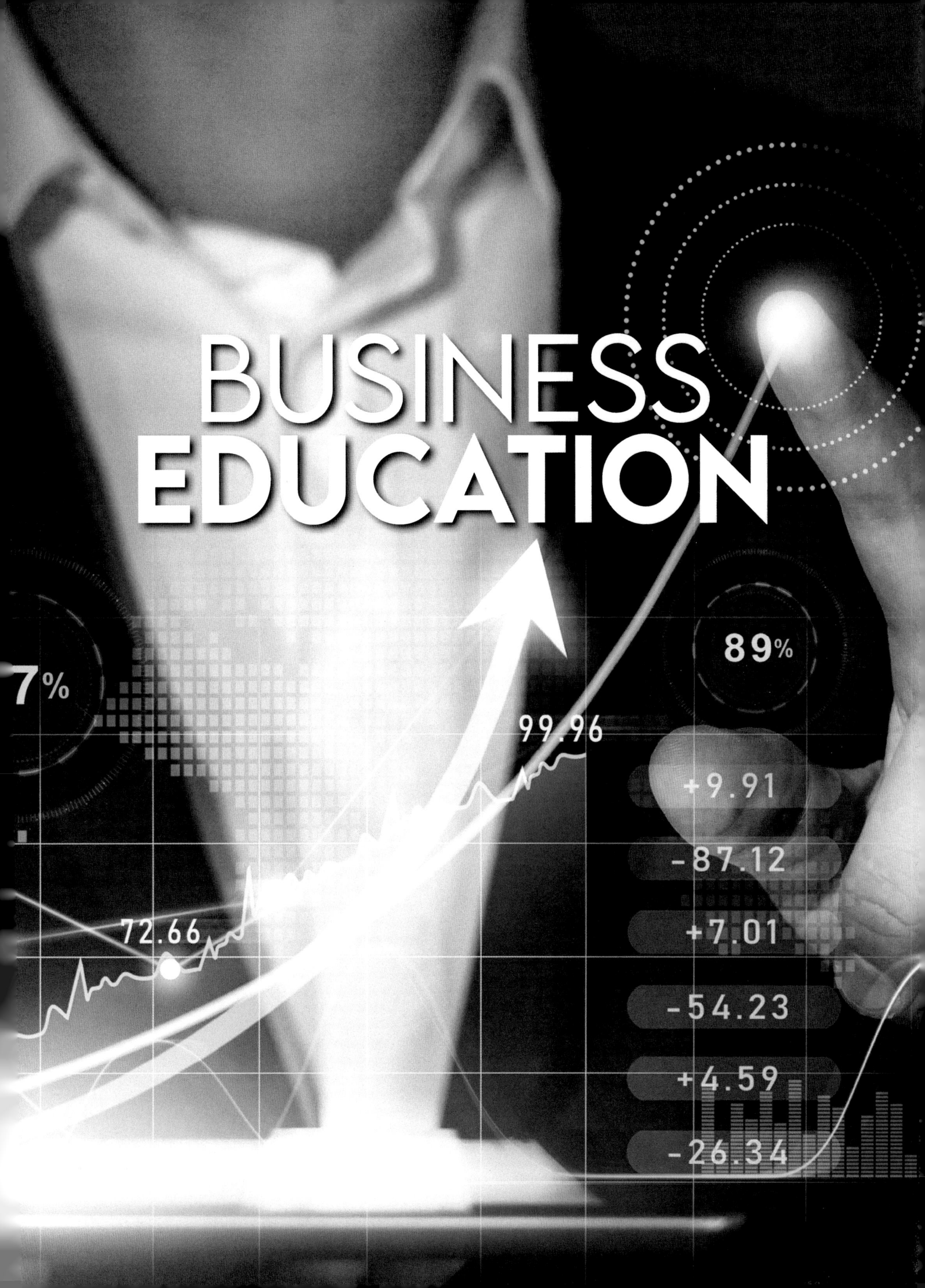

BUSINESS EDUCATION

7%

89%

99.96

+9.91

-87.12

+7.01

72.66

-54.23

+4.59

-26.34

THE OPPORTUNITY

- Network marketing in a professional direct sales system
- Not a copycat product – fully patented technology
- Uses a Binary system for a simple building strategy
- Only two legs – no more confusing stacking, just right or left
- Built in on-boarding system for customers and brand partners
- Earn while you learn system with effective building strategy
- Five ways to earn commission:
    1. Earn through product introductory bonuses
    2. Earn up to $25,000 per week on cycle bonuses
    3. Earn up to 25% on generation cycle matching bonuses
    4. Earn fast start bonuses on Premium package enrollments
    5. Earn through retail and preferred customer commissions

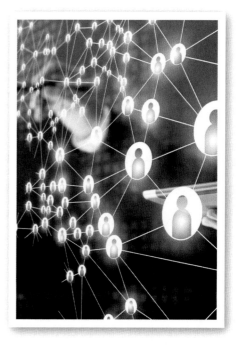

PRODUCT INTRODUCTORY BONUS EARNING EXAMPLE
To earn a minimum of $1000 USD per week on PIB alone.

Premium $405, Advanced $75, Core $35
- Enroll THREE Premium packages and get paid $1215 USD
- Enroll ONE Premium and EIGHT Advanced and get paid $1004
- Enroll ONE Premium, SIX Advanced, and FIVE Core and get paid $1030
- Enroll FOURTEEN Advanced and get paid $1050
- Enroll TWENTY-NINE Core and get paid $1015

CYCLE BONUS EARNING EXAMPLE
To earn a minimum of $1000 USD per week on Cycle Bonuses alone.
This example assumes you are Manager or above and would give you 20 cycles at $50 each for $1000 income for the week.
- Profit Leg (small leg) needs to be 6,600 points
- Power Leg (big leg) needs to be 13,200 points

BUILDER CHECKLIST

FIRST STEPS FOR BRAND PARTNERS
❏ Step 1: Complete "First Steps" checklist on page 6.

Finding Your URL and How to Switch Right or Left
❏ Step 2: Log into LifeWave.com and go to "Change Settings" at the top under your name
    ❏ Write out your URL _____ add /enrollment/packs
    ❏ What is your member number? _____
    ❏ What is your username? _____
    ❏ Locate "Build Left" and "Build Right" settings at the bottom

Understanding Your Organization
❏ Step 3: Go to Organization, then Binary Tree Viewer, and hover over your tile
    ❏ Note your Right Volume and Left Volume amounts. LV: _____ RV: _____
    ❏ If you have points on one side, how many and is it RV or LV? _____
    ❏ Which side of your tree has people you do not know?   Right   Left   None
    ❏ Based on the above information which side is your Power Leg? _____
        Power leg is the bigger leg, also called your outside leg
    ❏ Based on the above information which side is your Profit Leg? _____
        Profit leg is the smaller leg, also called your inside leg
    ❏ Cycle Bonuses: What two volume numbers allow you to cycle? _____ and _____
        Answer: 660BV on your power leg and 330BV on your profit leg

STEPS TO MANAGER
❏ Become a Brand Partner at Advanced or higher and maintain 110PV per month as active
❏ Based on the above Right-Left information, map out your first four enrollments
❏ Create a list of 100 people you know that could use this, then contact them
❏ Enroll four personally sponsored Brand Partner members (two on Left and two on Right)
❏ Ensure all your members stay ACTIVE at 55PV or more per rolling 31 day cycle
❏ Select Build Right or Build Left BEFORE you sign someone up
❏ To move someone, use Live Chat within five days of signing the person up

STEPS TO DIRECTOR
❏ Maintain Manager status
❏ Add one additional active personally sponsored (PS) Brand Partner to your Left and one on your Right
❏ Teach one PS on your Left how to get to Manager
❏ Teach one PS on your Right how to get to Manager

STEPS TO SENIOR DIRECTOR
❏ Maintain Director status
❏ Help two personally sponsored get to Director
❏ Get to 10,000 personal organizational volume

RESOURCES
www.LifeWave.com
www.LifeWaveSuccessLibrary.com
www.PatchEDU.com
www.YouTube.com/@PatchEDU

TERMINOLOGY

BASIC TERMINOLOGY
- ❏ LW = LifeWave
- ❏ PV = Personal Volume
- ❏ BV = Business Volume
- ❏ GVU = Group Volume Unilevel (same as GCV)
- ❏ GCV = Group Commissionable Volume
- ❏ LV = Left Volume (your left leg)
- ❏ RV = Right Volume (your right leg)
- ❏ PIB = Product Introductory Bonus
- ❏ BP = Brand Partner or Member
- ❏ PC = Preferred Customer
- ❏ PC+ = Preferred Customer Plus program (additional benefits)
- ❏ PS or PE = Personally Sponsored or Personally Enrolled: A person you enrolled personally
- ❏ Sponsor or Enroller: The person who enrolled you in LifeWave
- ❏ Personal Group: Your personal generations from your personally sponsored and down
- ❏ Generations: People you signed up, and people they signed up, etc. - like a family
- ❏ First Generation: A person you enrolled personally
- ❏ Second Generation: A person your personally sponsored has enrolled/sponsored
- ❏ Third Generation: A person your second generation has enrolled
- ❏ Upline: Those in leadership above you
- ❏ Downline: Those below you
- ❏ Binary Tree: two legs, one on the right and one on the left
- ❏ Enroller Tree: shows who you personally sponsored in order from left to right
- ❏ Rolling 31 Day PV: Your personal volume each 31 days based on your order date
- ❏ Trickle: For Premium or Maintenance Packs, your PV is spread out over several months
- ❏ Profit Leg: Your smaller leg (less points), also called your inside leg
- ❏ Power Leg: Your bigger leg (more points), also called your outside leg
- ❏ Inside Leg: If you are placed on someone's big leg, this is your smaller leg (less points)
- ❏ Outside Leg: If you are placed on someone's big leg, this is your bigger leg (more points)
- ❏ Cycle Bonus: $50 when your Profit Leg hits 330 BV and your Power Leg hits 660 BV

OTHER TERMS
- ❏ FDA = Food and Drug Administration
- ❏ FTC = Federal Trade Commission
- ❏ DSA = Direct Selling Association
- ❏ DSN = Direct Selling News
- ❏ Photobiomodulation = another word for phototherapy
- ❏ Attenuation = when a product becomes less effective due to overuse
- ❏ Proliferation = when cells rapidly reproduce or multiply

BUSINESS BASICS

HOW TO LOCATE YOUR PERSONAL URL
- Sign into your account at LifeWave.com
- Find your name at the top right and click on it
- Go under Change Settings
- Locate your Username under your email
- Add your username to the following URL to enroll a Brand Partner: LifeWave.com/_____/enrollment/packs

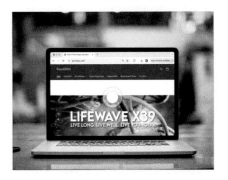

HOW TO SHARE X39 WITH OTHERS
- Share www.PatchEDU.com
- Patch or share X39 with three new people per day
- Follow up with three people per day
- Invite three people per day to an online meeting
- Use the InTouch LifeWave app to track people
- Share a video from YouTube

HOW TO ENROLL A FRIEND
- Give the person your personal URL: LifeWave.com/username/enrollment/packs
- Walk them through enrollment in person or on a call
- Send them the LifeWave Order Form (see page 61)
- Start at Core, Advanced, or Premium (share the benefits of a member/brand partner vs customer - see page 60)
- Always start with X39 and possibly add Aeon if needed
- Make sure they utilize one of these three options:
    1. Be on a monthly subscription
    2. Teach them the value of upgrading each month
    3. Buy a 3 or 6-month maintenance pack to stay active

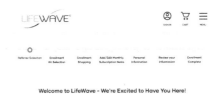

HOW TO ONBOARD YOUR NEW MEMBER
- Send them a welcome email with next steps
- Send them the Patch Manual
- Invite them to weekly online meetings
- Get them plugged in to the Facebook groups
- Follow up when they get their patches
- Share tips: increase water and use electrolytes
- Encourage them to use an alarm for patch on/off times
- Give tips from Patch Education on PatchEDU.com
- See suggestions on page 58 under Follow-up Notes

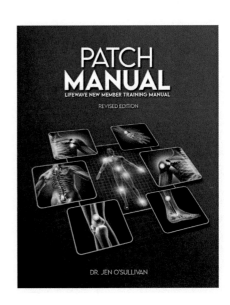

MINDSET TRAINING

SERVANT LEADERSHIP

The most successful fortune 500 companies are the ones where the CEO is willing to do the work with their employees. Consider any team you worked on in the past and what you wished the leader of that team would have done or been for the group. Superheroes are only heroes because they serve the people well. Be the leader you wish you had!

TRANSPARENCY

Be vulnerable with your team and share both your successes and your losses. When we fail at something there is always a lesson to be learned. You don't win some and lose some. Sometimes you win and sometimes you LEARN. Every loss is an opportunity to learn and grow. Transparency in your journey is key to building a team that trusts you and wants to run with you. Remember, a winner is just a loser who tried one more time.

KEEP IT SIMPLE

KISS is a fun acronym that means Keep It Simple Stupid. Sister or Silly work too! The point is, make sharing as simple as possible. People don't like "complicated" when it comes to network marketing, so the simpler the better! If you act like you know everything or seem too polished all the time, your team will feel like they will always fall short. Get them to a point where they say, "Wow, I can do that... and I probably can even do it BETTER!"

POSITIVE LANGUAGE

Your thoughts plus your feelings plus your actions equals your results. Using excuses when you fail or blame-shifting will not give you success. So much of our functional day-to-day actions are contrary to our confessional desires. If you want success, you must shift your language to that of a successful person. Negativity breeds negativity. Root out the cancers in your life. Also, check to make sure YOU are not the cancer in any group or community. Here are some positive language shifts:

"I want to be debt free" to "I want to be financially free"

"I'm terrible at selling" to "I love helping people"

"If you join me" to "When you join me"

"I'm too busy" to "I get stuff done"

"I'm broke" to "Other people have my money and it will come to me soon."

"Money doesn't grow on trees" to "We have money and we are wise in how we use it"

"Money is the root of all evil" to "Money is a God-given tool to help more people"

IDENTITY SHIFTING

Goal setting has its place, but ultimately setting goals is useless without one key change. You will never obtain your goal until you shift your identity. If your goal is to make $10,000 per week, but your functional identity is that of a couch potato, it will be pretty impossible to reach your goal. If, on the other hand, you are a couch potato who wants to reach the $10,000 per week goal, all you need to do is ask yourself, "How does the $10,000 per week person run their business and life?" I bet those people are pretty organized, dedicated, and their couch is seldom used. It is the same with any goal. If you want to be fit and at your goal body weight, shift your identity to a fit person. Consistently ask yourself, "What would a fit person order?" or "Would a fit person take the stairs or the elevator?" or "What type of lifestyle does a fit person have?" and then do those things!

TRAINING GUIDE

EDUCATION
- ❏ Start Here: www.PatchEDU.com
- ❏ Patch Instructions: www.LifeWaveSuccessLibrary.com
- ❏ Download the InTouch LifeWave app
- ❏ YouTube Trainings: www.YouTube.com/@PatchEDU
- ❏ Manual, brochures, and downloads: www.PatchEDU.com
- ❏ Product Education Series: https://tinyurl.com/X39product
- ❏ Business Training Series: https://tinyurl.com/X39business
- ❏ Inventor's Explanation: https://youtu.be/JwpWNcqtjCo (18 minutes)
- ❏ Horses Don't Lie: https://youtu.be/8sw4rAHwzhc (4 minutes)

BUSINESS
- ❏ Patch or introduce X39 to three people per day
- ❏ Follow up with three people per day
- ❏ Invite three people per day to an online training and opportunity introduction
- ❏ Invite 1-3 entrepreneurs to an online business introduction event

ONLINE TRAINING
- ❏ Attend at least two online meetings per week – one on product and one on business
- ❏ Host your own online meeting at least once per week. Practice, practice, practice!

SOCIAL MEDIA ACTIVITY
- ❏ Know your people and post accordingly – what is their age, gender, likes, and hobbies
- ❏ Post about things people have opinions on, not photos of your food
- ❏ Post a "curiosity" post – ask something that gets your audience to question what it is
- ❏ Post on social media using a 5/1 method. Five social posts, then one about X39
- ❏ Never mention X39 outright. Post about a testimony and leave out X39 or Lifewave
- ❏ Actively comment on other comments right away – do not mention X39
- ❏ Follow up with those who comment in a private message
- ❏ Invite friends via private message to online meetings and X39 Lifewave Education group
- ❏ Drip on friends who have shown interest with short videos, texts, and social engagement
- ❏ Share PatchEDU.com and invite them to watch the first two short videos

WARM MARKET
- ❏ Develop a list of your warm market – start with 100 to 300 people – add to it weekly
- ❏ Create a follow-up schedule with your people so you can track what you sent them
- ❏ Use InTouch LifeWave app or a simple spreadsheet for tracking

FOLLOW UP STRATEGIES
- ❏ Invite to an online meeting
- ❏ Invite to a live meeting or event
- ❏ Invite to the open education group on Facebook called Patch EDU
- ❏ Share the patch basics on one of the regular patches
- ❏ Ask if they are having any detox and remind them about water and electrolytes
- ❏ Share your favorite electrolyte product
- ❏ Ask to hear their testimony to date

THE FOUR BELIEFS

BELIEF IN THE PRODUCT
In order to get others passionate about something, you must be passionate about it. You must have 100% unwavering belief in the patches you sell in order to sell them. People will buy your passion about the patches, before they buy the patches themselves. Your tone matters just as much as your words. Get excited about what you have to offer because no one else on the planet offers them! X39 is unlike anything else and offers some of the most profound and life-changing benefits to anyone with a heartbeat. Take a look at the front of this Manual for all the information on these incredible patches!

BELIEF IN THE COMPANY
Any company you align yourself with has their own set of ethics, philosophies, and standards by which they operate. These standards should closely align with your own. Take some time to listen to the founder, David Schmidt, through the various trainings available online. Read about how LifeWave began on the LifeWave.com website. Read "The Story of X39" by David Schmidt for a great perspective on how the X39 came to be at tinyurl.com/X39-story and then get excited about the massive gift LifeWave has given you not only for your personal health, but financial health too!

BELIEF IN THE INDUSTRY
The network marketing or direct sales industry is an incredibly lucrative industry. As of a 2022 Direct Selling Association release, the direct selling industry generates $40.5 billion in sales and has over 6.7 million entrepreneurs selling on a part-time or full-time basis. There are many names for the industry such as direct sales, network marketing, social selling, referral marketing, affiliate marketing, and multilevel marketing (MLM), with the latter often coming with preconceived negative notions. Some people think all direct sales companies are pyramid schemes. All forms of pyramid schemes are illegal. Large corporations have more of a pyramid shape than direct sales companies do. One person at the top makes all the money with hundreds of thousands of workers at the bottom making minimum wage. With direct sales, there is no glass ceiling, and instead of the company paying 60% or more on their marketing budget, they give that to the brand partners who are selling their product. Most direct sales companies only pay 40-50% of their profits to their brand partners. LifeWave pays its brand partners in the field a generous 60%. The added bonus of shopping with trusted friends and helping put food on their table is also something to consider, rather than lining the pockets of big industry.

BELIEF IN YOURSELF
Belief in yourself is the most important belief of all four. This is the belief that will allow you to either succeed or fail. Many people were brought up in a world of "I can't" or "I'm afraid." Most of us are full of excuses as to why we are not good enough, but when it comes right down to it, 99% of the time you can succeed if you only get out of your own way. Network marketing is WORK, but it is extremely rewarding when you do it right. If someone were told they had to work 90 hours a week for two years and they were guaranteed a $400,000 salary, they would most likely go for it. Instead people work a dreary 8am to 6pm job and can barely make ends meet. As of 2024, the average annual salary in the USA is just over $60,000. What would an extra $400,000 do for you? Who could you bless? What type of time freedom would you have? What type of choice freedom would you have? To place this in perspective, the average Senior Presidential Director with LifeWave makes just under $400,000 per year and it takes an average of two years to get to that rank (see the 2023 LifeWave Income Disclosure on page 42). Are you ready to start believing in yourself?

THE LIVE EVENT

STEP ONE: INVITES
- Invite four times the amount of people you would like to attend. For 10 people, invite 40.
- Personally invite each person one to two weeks prior to the event as a "save the date".
- Invite people in person or over the phone. It is important to not send a group text or email.
- When someone confirms their attendance, give them the basics such as time and location. Leave out pertinent information. This will give you reasons to connect with them later as reminders.

STEP TWO: CONNECTION POINTS
- One week before the event, contact each person attending and ask if they can help you with the event. Examples: come early to help set up, come early to help welcome guests at the door, bring extra folding chairs, ask them to bring their famous dip, you get the idea. Ask every single attendee to help in some way. Play to their strengths such as, "Lisa, you are so welcoming and loving. Would you be willing to help greet guests at the door for the party?" This ensures everyone will attend as each person is responsible for something specific. It keeps your guests accountable to show up.
- Four days before the event, ask if they have any friends they would like to invite.
- Two days before, share your address. If they know it already, say it is for friends they want to invite.
- One day before, thank them for helping and give any details that pertain to their area of service.
- The day of, let them know your door will be unlocked and to please come in when they arrive (assuming your neighborhood is safe and/or this is even an option in your area.)

STEP THREE: THE PATCH PARTY, EVENT, OR CLASS
There are many ways to approach a patch party, event, or class. Lean into your strengths and do something fun! Have some inexpensive party gifts to give out, such as electrolyte sticks, packs of sea salt, a patch, or even a drawing to win a larger prize depending on the size of your event. Your event, party, or class should be no longer than 90 minutes under normal circumstances.
1. Have a pre-party get together in the kitchen with drinks and light snacks. Don't overdo it with decorations and a lot of food. You want it to be duplicatable in the minds of your guests.
2. Gather everyone into your main room for the info session. This should start around 15 minutes in.
3. Welcome everyone and thank them for coming, then show the 2-minute phototherapy video.
4. Share your testimony in 3-5 minutes. Do not make this any longer. Short and sweet.
5. Share about the X39 patch. The education part should take 15-20 minutes. Hand out a brochure*. Follow one of the presentations on PatchEDU.com. Note: use the X39 presentation first. During the presentation, show the power of the patches by patching a guest.
6. Ask those who have tried X39 to share their testimony. If none, share some you have heard about.
7. Go over the various packages and buy-in options. Remind them of the money-back guarantee.
8. Share the opportunity portion of the presentation. This portion should take 10-15 minutes.
9. Don't forget to laugh and have fun. Talk about any common issues some people may have.
10. ASK FOR THE SALE! "Who is ready to get healthy with X39? Let's enroll you now!" Pass out an enrollment form and a pen to everyone there. Offer an incentive to those who enroll at the event.

STEP FOUR: FOLLOW-UP
Follow-up with everyone who attended. Thank them for coming. Share your excitement with those who enrolled. Give them some onboarding material such as this Patch Manual. Ask more questions to those who did not enroll. Your goal is to help them get healthy!

STEP FIVE: PRACTICE, PRACTICE, PRACTICE!
The more you host parties, events, and classes, the better you will become at presenting, and the easier and more fun they will be for both you and your guests. For any event you host, invite everyone, including those who are already on your team under you. The more the merrier!

*Brochures and slide presentations available at PatchEDU.com

GETTING PAID

ELIGIBILITY

You will be notified by LifeWave once you are eligible to set up I-Payout, so please be patient. Depending on when you made your first sale, it could be up to three full weeks before you have access to your money. Once you make your first sale, the PIB (Product Introductory Bonus) and any additional commissions will be available on Tuesday, two weeks after the week pay period ending on Sunday the week of the sale.

As an example, if you sell something on a Monday, you will not be able to access that money for three weeks and one day. If you sell something on a Sunday, you will not be able to access that commission for two weeks and two days.

I-PAYOUT

❏ Log into your LifeWave account at LifeWave.com
❏ Click the blue PAY PORTAL link under Your Commissions tile on the left
❏ Click the blue LOGIN TO I-PAYOUT link
❏ Once you are eligible to withdraw funds, you will be able to set up I-PAYOUT

METHODS OF PAYMENT

❏ Set up a bank account to transfer your money to
❏ Set up a wire profile to wire transfer
❏ Request a physical check
❏ Order a prepaid MasterCard credit card
❏ Set up Auto Withdrawal to pay you on a certain day of the month or to get payment once a specific amount has been reached that you decide upon

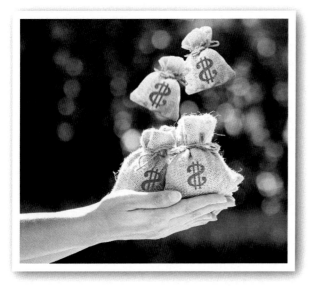

Note: I-Payout has a limit of $5,000 weekly. To increase this amount to $10,000 per week you must submit to LifeWave corporate your government issued ID (driver's license or passport) and a proof of address such as a utility bill.

International Member Note: If you choose the prepaid credit card, you may use this card to pay for your orders on your account. This is helpful for those of you in international markets as your payment will be in USD and your purchases will be in USD. You will not have to deal with or worry about the exchange rate.

COMMISSIONS

PIB: PRODUCT INTRODUCTORY BONUS

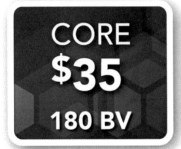
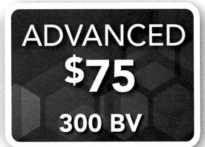
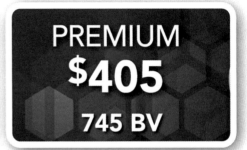

CORE
$35
180 BV

ADVANCED
$75
300 BV

PREMIUM
$405
745 BV

RETAIL & PREFERRED CUSTOMER COMMISSIONS

RETAIL CUSTOMER

$50 profit and 77 BV on X39 sleeve for $149.95

PREFERRED CUSTOMER

$20 profit and 43 BV on X39 sleeve for $99.95

PC+ CUSTOMER

$20 profit and 43 BV when they purchase an X39 sleeve for $99.95

BONUS: *For each customer a PC+ person brings in, you get the $20 profit on each of their orders! When they sign up three people, you get $60 and they get free product!*

CYCLE BONUSES

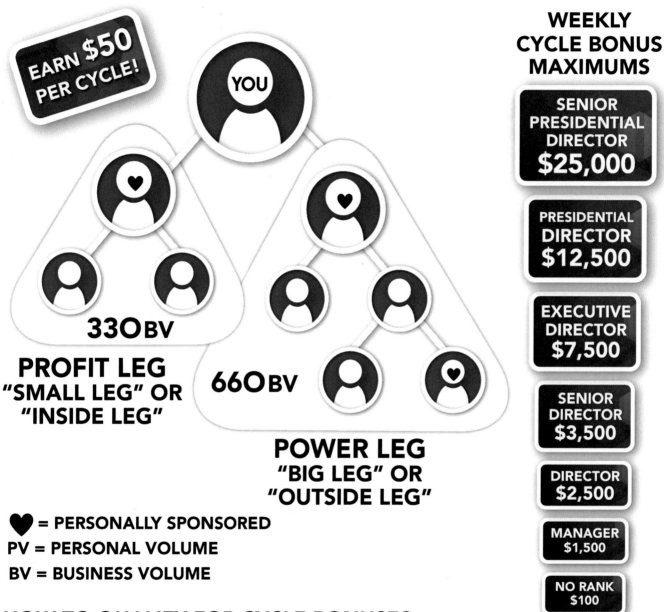

EARN $50 PER CYCLE!

YOU

330 BV

PROFIT LEG
"SMALL LEG" OR "INSIDE LEG"

660 BV

POWER LEG
"BIG LEG" OR "OUTSIDE LEG"

WEEKLY CYCLE BONUS MAXIMUMS

SENIOR PRESIDENTIAL DIRECTOR	$25,000
PRESIDENTIAL DIRECTOR	$12,500
EXECUTIVE DIRECTOR	$7,500
SENIOR DIRECTOR	$3,500
DIRECTOR	$2,500
MANAGER	$1,500
NO RANK	$100

♥ = PERSONALLY SPONSORED
PV = PERSONAL VOLUME
BV = BUSINESS VOLUME

HOW TO QUALIFY FOR CYCLE BONUSES

1. Stay active with 55PV+ per rolling 31 day cycle
2. Have one or more personally sponsored, active Brand Partners on each leg
3. Have 330BV+ on your Profit leg and 660BV+ on your Power leg
Once a cycle is redeemed, that volume is subtracted from your total volume.

GENERATION PAY

25% **1ST GENERATION**
YOUR PERSONALLY SPONSORED

EARNINGS:
Earn 25% on your personally sponsored cycle bonuses

QUALIFICATIONS:
Active Manager Status

GET PAID ON YOUR PERSONALLY SPONSORED CYCLE BONUSES

20% **2ND GENERATION**
THOSE ENROLLED BY YOUR 1ST GEN.

EARNINGS:
Earn 20% on your second generation cycle bonuses

QUALIFICATIONS:
1. Active Manager Status
2. *Must have a minimum of six cycles in weekly earnings*

GENERATION MATCHING IS A LARGE PART OF YOUR PAY CHECK ON MATURE TEAMS

20% **3RD GENERATION**
THOSE ENROLLED BY YOUR 2ND GEN.

EARNINGS:
Earn 20% on your third generation cycle bonuses

QUALIFICATIONS:
1. Active Manager Status
2. *Must have a minimum of ten cycles in weekly earnings*
3. *Each leg has 3 active BPs*
4. *One manager earning 2nd gen. matching on each leg*

MANAGER

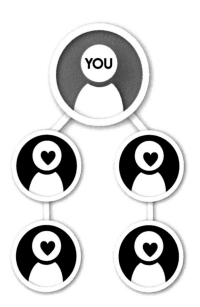

QUALIFICATIONS

- Lifetime 300PV+ or purchase Advanced or Premium
- Active status at 110PV or more in 31 day period
- Four active (55PV+) personally sponsored Brand Partners – two on Left and two on Right

YOUR GOAL

- Become a Manager Making Machine!

- Teach one personally sponsored member on each side how to become Manager

- Continue to focus ONLY on helping people below you become Manager!

DIRECTOR

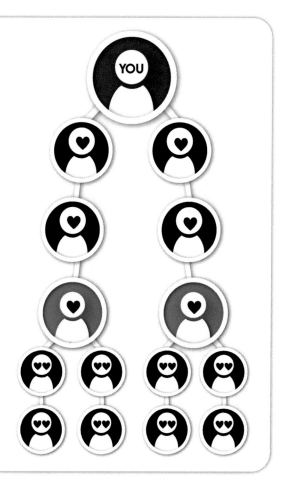

QUALIFICATIONS

- Lifetime 300PV+ or purchase Advanced or Premium
- Active status at 110PV or more in 31 day period
- Six active (55PV+) personally sponsored (PS) Brand Partners – three on Left and three on Right
- One personally sponsored Manager on your Left
- One personally sponsored Manager on your Right

YOUR GOAL

- Continue to make Managers!
- Teach your PS to teach others to make Managers

BECOME A MANAGER MAKING MACHINE!

SENIOR DIRECTOR

QUALIFICATIONS
- Lifetime 300PV+ or purchase Advanced or Premium
- Active status at 110PV or more in 31 day period
- Six active (55PV+) personally sponsored (PS) Brand Partners – three on Left and three on Right
- Have a Manager or higher on each leg (Directors count)
- Two personally sponsored Directors or higher
- **10,000+ in GVU**

YOUR GOAL
- Continue to make Managers!
- Teach your PS to teach others to make Managers
- Focus on building your volume moving forward!

DIRECTORS CAN BE ON THE SAME LEG

10,000+ in GVU

ICON KEY
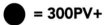 ● = 300PV+
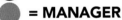 ● = MANAGER
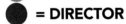 ● = DIRECTOR
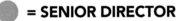 ● = SENIOR DIRECTOR
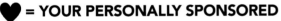 ♥ = YOUR PERSONALLY SPONSORED
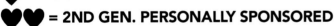 ♥♥ = 2ND GEN. PERSONALLY SPONSORED

BP = BRAND PARTNER
PV = PERSONAL VOLUME
PS = PERSONALLY SPONSORED
GVU = GROUP VOLUME UNILEVEL

EXECUTIVE DIRECTOR

300PV or more lifetime and active status at 110PV or more each month

Six active PS BPs
Three on each side

Two Personally Sponsored Directors or higher

50,000+ in GVU

PRESIDENTIAL DIRECTOR

300PV or more lifetime and active status at 110PV or more each month

Six active PS BPs
Three on each side

Two Personally Sponsored Directors or higher

100,000+ in GVU

SENIOR PRESIDENTIAL DIRECTOR

300PV or more lifetime and active status at 110PV or more each month

Six active PS BPs
Three on each side

Two Personally Sponsored Directors or higher

200,000+ in GVU

BRAND PARTNER TRACKER
LEFT LEG MAIN LEADERS

NAME_____ City/State/Country_____

ID# _____ Date Enrolled _____ Birthday _____

Cell Phone _____ Email _____

Generation_____ **Rank & Date** M_____ D_____ SD_____ ED_____ PD_____ SPD_____

Package ❑ CORE (buy date)_____ ❑ ADVANCED (buy date)_____ ❑ PREMIUM (buy date)_____

Sleeves ❑ X39 ❑ X49 ❑ Aeon ❑ Glut ❑ Carn ❑ SP6 ❑ AV ❑ Ice ❑ EE ❑ SN

Subscription ❑ Maintenance ❑ Monthly **Monthly Order Date** _____ PV _____

Follow-up Notes ❑ Onboarding email ❑ In team groups ❑ Invite to Zooms
❑ Patch Manual order ❑ X39 Health Tracker ❑ Web walk-through ❑ Share opportunity
❑ Patch arrival call/text ❑ 24-hour follow-up ❑ Water checkup ❑ 12/12 hr. follow-up
❑ 3-day follow-up (detox, water, electrolytes) ❑ Share experience ❑ Share with others

Additional Notes _____

NAME_____ City/State/Country_____

ID# _____ Date Enrolled _____ Birthday _____

Cell Phone _____ Email _____

Generation_____ **Rank & Date** M_____ D_____ SD_____ ED_____ PD_____ SPD_____

Package ❑ CORE (buy date)_____ ❑ ADVANCED (buy date)_____ ❑ PREMIUM (buy date)_____

Sleeves ❑ X39 ❑ X49 ❑ Aeon ❑ Glut ❑ Carn ❑ SP6 ❑ AV ❑ Ice ❑ EE ❑ SN

Subscription ❑ Maintenance ❑ Monthly **Monthly Order Date** _____ PV _____

Follow-up Notes ❑ Onboarding email ❑ In team groups ❑ Invite to Zooms
❑ Patch Manual order ❑ X39 Health Tracker ❑ Web walk-through ❑ Share opportunity
❑ Patch arrival call/text ❑ 24-hour follow-up ❑ Water checkup ❑ 12/12 hr. follow-up
❑ 3-day follow-up (detox, water, electrolytes) ❑ Share experience ❑ Share with others

Additional Notes _____

NAME_____ City/State/Country_____

ID# _____ Date Enrolled _____ Birthday _____

Cell Phone _____ Email _____

Generation_____ **Rank & Date** M_____ D_____ SD_____ ED_____ PD_____ SPD_____

Package ❑ CORE (buy date)_____ ❑ ADVANCED (buy date)_____ ❑ PREMIUM (buy date)_____

Sleeves ❑ X39 ❑ X49 ❑ Aeon ❑ Glut ❑ Carn ❑ SP6 ❑ AV ❑ Ice ❑ EE ❑ SN

Subscription ❑ Maintenance ❑ Monthly **Monthly Order Date** _____ PV _____

Follow-up Notes ❑ Onboarding email ❑ In team groups ❑ Invite to Zooms
❑ Patch Manual order ❑ X39 Health Tracker ❑ Web walk-through ❑ Share opportunity
❑ Patch arrival call/text ❑ 24-hour follow-up ❑ Water checkup ❑ 12/12 hr. follow-up
❑ 3-day follow-up (detox, water, electrolytes) ❑ Share experience ❑ Share with others

Additional Notes _____

RIGHT LEG MAIN LEADERS

NAME_____ City/State/Country_____

ID# _____ Date Enrolled _____ Birthday _____

Cell Phone _____ Email _____

Generation_____ **Rank & Date** M_____ D_____ SD_____ ED_____ PD_____ SPD_____

Package ❏ CORE (buy date)_____ ❏ ADVANCED (buy date)_____ ❏ PREMIUM (buy date)_____

Sleeves ❏ X39 ❏ X49 ❏ Aeon ❏ Glut ❏ Carn ❏ SP6 ❏ AV ❏ Ice ❏ EE ❏ SN

Subscription ❏ Maintenance ❏ Monthly **Monthly Order Date** _____ PV _____

Follow-up Notes
❏ Onboarding email ❏ In team groups ❏ Invite to Zooms
❏ Patch Manual order ❏ X39 Health Tracker ❏ Web walk-through ❏ Share opportunity
❏ Patch arrival call/text ❏ 24-hour follow-up ❏ Water checkup ❏ 12/12 hr. follow-up
❏ 3-day follow-up (detox, water, electrolytes) ❏ Share experience ❏ Share with others

Additional Notes _____

NAME_____ City/State/Country_____

ID# _____ Date Enrolled _____ Birthday _____

Cell Phone _____ Email _____

Generation_____ **Rank & Date** M_____ D_____ SD_____ ED_____ PD_____ SPD_____

Package ❏ CORE (buy date)_____ ❏ ADVANCED (buy date)_____ ❏ PREMIUM (buy date)_____

Sleeves ❏ X39 ❏ X49 ❏ Aeon ❏ Glut ❏ Carn ❏ SP6 ❏ AV ❏ Ice ❏ EE ❏ SN

Subscription ❏ Maintenance ❏ Monthly **Monthly Order Date** _____ PV _____

Follow-up Notes
❏ Onboarding email ❏ In team groups ❏ Invite to Zooms
❏ Patch Manual order ❏ X39 Health Tracker ❏ Web walk-through ❏ Share opportunity
❏ Patch arrival call/text ❏ 24-hour follow-up ❏ Water checkup ❏ 12/12 hr. follow-up
❏ 3-day follow-up (detox, water, electrolytes) ❏ Share experience ❏ Share with others

Additional Notes _____

NAME_____ City/State/Country_____

ID# _____ Date Enrolled _____ Birthday _____

Cell Phone _____ Email _____

Generation_____ **Rank & Date** M_____ D_____ SD_____ ED_____ PD_____ SPD_____

Package ❏ CORE (buy date)_____ ❏ ADVANCED (buy date)_____ ❏ PREMIUM (buy date)_____

Sleeves ❏ X39 ❏ X49 ❏ Aeon ❏ Glut ❏ Carn ❏ SP6 ❏ AV ❏ Ice ❏ EE ❏ SN

Subscription ❏ Maintenance ❏ Monthly **Monthly Order Date** _____ PV _____

Follow-up Notes
❏ Onboarding email ❏ In team groups ❏ Invite to Zooms
❏ Patch Manual order ❏ X39 Health Tracker ❏ Web walk-through ❏ Share opportunity
❏ Patch arrival call/text ❏ 24-hour follow-up ❏ Water checkup ❏ 12/12 hr. follow-up
❏ 3-day follow-up (detox, water, electrolytes) ❏ Share experience ❏ Share with others

Additional Notes _____

MEMBER DISCOUNTS

PATCHEDU.COM

All pricing on this page is in USD. When you join as a member (also called a Brand Partner) there are several perks you get that you will not get when joining as a Preferred Customer or Preferred Customer Plus. The below package savings are based on membership pricing. If you join as a Preferred Customer, the wholesale pricing amount would apply to you.

MEMBERSHIP & BRAND PARTNER BENEFITS

- ❏ Discounted Membership packages – larger packages equal deeper discounts
- ❏ Access to Upgrade packages – start at one package, then upgrade by paying the difference
- ❏ Access to discounted Maintenance packages –order 3 or 6 month packs and save on shipping plus the larger the pack, the greater the additional discount you receive
- ❏ Get up to 12 months to consider sharing LifeWave with friends and family to make commissions
Stay active monthly at 55 BV and keep building your points for potential cycle bonuses
Once you rank to Manager, you will need 110 PV monthly to stay active and keep your points

X39 ONLY PACKS

The X39 patch is LifeWave's foundational health patch. Buying only X39 in your starter pack ensures you get the very best pricing. Adding Aeon can help enhance the performance of X39 when you have extra stress or inflammation in your life. Choose the best pack for your needs!

Core Package
Three X39 sleeves
30 patches per sleeve
$295 pack price
$98.33 per X39 sleeve

Advanced Package
Six X39 sleeves
30 patches per sleeve
$535 pack price
$89.17 per X39 sleeve

Premium Package
20 X39 sleeves
30 patches per sleeve
$1750 pack price
$87.50 per X39 sleeve

MEMBERSHIP SAVES YOU OVER 43% ON WHOLESALE WITH THE PREMIUM PACK

CORE PACKAGE $295
$459.80 retail
$364.80 wholesale
Based on two X39 and two Aeon

RETAIL		WHOLESALE	
1 X39	$149.95	1 X39	$99.95
1 X39	$149.95	1 X39	$99.95
1 Aeon	$79.95	1 Aeon	$69.95
1 Aeon	$79.95	1 Aeon	$69.95
Fee*	$0	Fee*	$25.00
Total	$459.80	Total	$364.80
Core	$295.00	Core	$295.00
Savings	$164.80	Savings	$69.80

ADVANCED PACKAGE $535
$919.60 retail
$704.60 wholesale
Based on four X39 and four Aeon

RETAIL		WHOLESALE	
1 X39	$149.95	1 X39	$99.95
1 X39	$149.95	1 X39	$99.95
1 X39	$149.95	1 X39	$99.95
1 X39	$149.95	1 X39	$99.95
1 Aeon	$79.95	1 Aeon	$69.95
1 Aeon	$79.95	1 Aeon	$69.95
1 Aeon	$79.95	1 Aeon	$69.95
1 Aeon	$79.95	1 Aeon	$69.95
Fee*	$0	Fee*	$25.00
Total	$919.60	Total	$704.60
Advanced	$535.00	Advanced	$535.00
Savings	$384.60	Savings	$169.60

* "Fee" means the membership fee paid to get wholesale pricing. Retail orders do not have a membership fee. The membership fee is only deducted once a Core or higher package is purchased. The annual membership fee renewal after 12 months is $25 for active Brand Partners/members.

PREMIUM PACK $1750
$3088.55 retail
$2313.60 wholesale
10 X39, 10 Aeon, 1 X49, and 8 others

RETAIL		WHOLESALE	
1 X39	$149.95	1 X39	$99.95
1 X39	$149.95	1 X39	$99.95
1 X39	$149.95	1 X39	$99.95
1 X39	$149.95	1 X39	$99.95
1 X39	$149.95	1 X39	$99.95
1 X39	$149.95	1 X39	$99.95
1 X39	$149.95	1 X39	$99.95
1 X39	$149.95	1 X39	$99.95
1 X39	$149.95	1 X39	$99.95
1 X39	$149.95	1 X39	$99.95
1 Aeon	$79.95	1 Aeon	$69.95
1 Aeon	$79.95	1 Aeon	$69.95
1 Aeon	$79.95	1 Aeon	$69.95
1 Aeon	$79.95	1 Aeon	$69.95
1 Aeon	$79.95	1 Aeon	$69.95
1 Aeon	$79.95	1 Aeon	$69.95
1 Aeon	$79.95	1 Aeon	$69.95
1 Aeon	$79.95	1 Aeon	$69.95
1 Aeon	$79.95	1 Aeon	$69.95
1 Aeon	$79.95	1 Aeon	$69.95
1 X49	$149.95	1 X49	$99.95
1 Glut	$79.95	1 Glut	$69.95
1 Carn	$79.95	1 Carn	$69.95
1 Alavida	$79.95	1 Alavida	$69.95
1 Alavida	$79.95	1 Alavida	$69.95
1 IceWave	$79.95	1 IceWave	$69.95
1 Energy	$79.95	1 Energy	$69.95
1 Silent	$79.95	1 Silent	$69.95
1 SP6	$79.95	1 SP6	$69.95
Fee*	$0	Fee*	$25.00
Total	$3088.55	Total	$2383.55
Premium	$1750.00	Premium	$1750.00
Savings	$1338.55	Savings	$633.55

LIFEWAVE ORDER FORM

PATCHEDU.COM

EACH SLEEVE CONTAINS 30 PATCHES, UNLESS OTHERWISE NOTED
APPLY PATCHES TO CLEAN, DRY SKIN AND WEAR FOR 12 HOURS. WEAR A NEW PATCH DAILY.

☐ PREMIUM
FOR LARGE FAMILIES OR THE SERIOUS ENTREPRENEUR

$1750 USD
THREE MONTHS ACTIVE STATUS
30 DAY GUARANTEE
(745 POINTS)

20 SLEEVES X39
OR CREATE YOUR CUSTOM ORDER TO EQUAL **40 CREDITS** – X39 & X49 EACH COUNT AS TWO CREDITS, ALL OTHER SLEEVES COUNT AS ONE

EXAMPLE CUSTOM ORDER
10 SLEEVES X39 (LONGEVITY/REPAIR)
10 SLEEVES AEON (STRESS/PAIN)
1 SLEEVE X49 (ATHLETES/BONE/EMF)
2 SLEEVES ALAVIDA (SKIN/SLEEP)
1 SLEEVE GLUTATHIONE (DETOX)
1 SLEEVE CARNOSINE (BRAIN)
1 SLEEVE ICEWAVE* (PAIN)
1 SLEEVE ENERGY ENHANCER*
1 SLEEVE SILENT NIGHTS (SLEEP)
1 SLEEVE SP6 (CRAVINGS/HORMONES)
* CONTAINS A 15 DAY SUPPLY

☐ ADVANCED
FOR MEDIUM SIZED FAMILIES OR THE NEW BUSINESS BUILDER

$535 USD
30 DAY GUARANTEE
(300 POINTS)

6 SLEEVES X39
OR CREATE YOUR CUSTOM ORDER TO EQUAL **12 CREDITS** – X39 & X49 EACH COUNT AS TWO CREDITS, ALL OTHER SLEEVES COUNT AS ONE

EXAMPLE CUSTOM ORDER
4 SLEEVES X39 AND
4 SLEEVES AEON

(MONEY BACK 30 DAY GUARANTEE seal)

☐ CORE
FOR INDIVIDUALS & COUPLES OR TO GET STARTED SLOWER

$295 USD
30 DAY GUARANTEE
(180 POINTS)

3 SLEEVES X39
OR CREATE YOUR CUSTOM ORDER TO EQUAL **6 CREDITS** – X39 & X49 EACH COUNT AS TWO CREDITS, ALL OTHER SLEEVES COUNT AS ONE

EXAMPLE CUSTOM ORDER
2 SLEEVES X39 AND
2 SLEEVES AEON

☐ **RETAIL:** ONE SLEEVE X39 = $149⁹⁵USD • NO MEMBERSHIP FEE OR AUTOSHIP • 90 DAY GUARANTEE

☐ **WHOLESALE:** ONE SLEEVE X39 = $99⁹⁵USD • $25 MEMBERSHIP FEE • 30 DAY GUARANTEE

☐ **PC:** PREFERRED CUSTOMER - WHOLESALE PRICING • NO ACCESS TO DEEPER DISCOUNTS ON STARTER PACKAGES
ONE SLEEVE X39 = $99⁹⁵USD • NO MEMBERSHIP FEE • ON AUTOSHIP • 90 DAY GUARANTEE

☐ **PC+:** PREFERRED CUSTOMER PLUS - WHOLESALE PRICING • FREE SAMPLES • NO ACCESS TO DISCOUNTS ON PACKAGES
ONE SLEEVE X39 = $99⁹⁵USD • $19.95 MEMBERSHIP FEE • ON AUTOSHIP • 90 DAY GUARANTEE

MONTHLY SUBSCRIPTION OPTIONS (MAY CUSTOMIZE AND CANCEL AT ANYTIME)

☐ TWO SLEEVES OF X39 $199⁹⁰USD PER MONTH (154 PV)	☐ ONE SLEEVE OF X39 $99⁹⁵USD PER MONTH (77 PV)	☐ ONE SLEEVE OF AEON $69⁹⁵USD PER MONTH (55 PV)

MEMBER INFORMATION

FIRST AND LAST NAME	MOBILE PHONE
ADDRESS	EMAIL
CITY, STATE, ZIP	DATE OF BIRTH

YOUR DESIRED USER NAME LifeWave.com/	PASSWORD	SPONSOR'S NAME OR ID NUMBER

PAYMENT INFORMATION

☐ BILLING ADDRESS SAME AS SHIPPING

NAME ON CREDIT CARD	BILLING ADDRESS IF DIFFERENT THAN ABOVE	
CARD NUMBER	EXPIRATION MONTH/YEAR	CVV CODE
SIGNATURE	DATE	

Health, Fitness & Dieting › Reference
Education & Teaching › Studying & Workbooks › Study Guides
Business & Money › Marketing & Sales › Sales & Selling › General

PATCH MANUAL

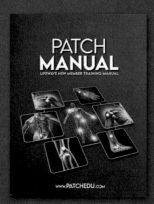

This Patch Manual is your go-to resource for everything pertaining to LifeWave® patches and the popular X39® patch. LifeWave patches are a unique and innovative technology that combines proven science and results that empower you to obtain optimal health without the use of invasive procedures or supplements that can be hard on your liver.

The most important patch is called X39 and is the foundation to optimal health. Proper use of X39 has been proven to significantly increase human GHK-Cu copper peptide in the body. By increasing the human production of GHK-Cu, it has been proven to also increase healthy stem cell activity. Wear X39 for 12 hours per day, giving yourself a 12 hour break before applying a new patch. Do this for a minimum of 6-12 months, and then continue daily use to maintain your health benefits. Use the health tracker in the Patch Manual to determine your starting points and progress. Get regular doctor check-ups at 6 and 12 months to track any internal progress you may not have noticed.

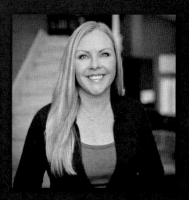

About the Author: Dr. Jen O'Sullivan is a Board Certified Doctor of Naturopathy, a Certified Master Herbalist, a Certified French Medicinal Aromatherapist, and a Licensed Ecclesiastical Holistic Practitioner. She works with her clients from a holistic, whole-body perspective focusing on the foundations of health and wellness both spiritually and physically. Dr. Jen is one of the most trusted and reliable educators in the complementary and alternative medicine field because she is known for her helpful, logical, and efficacious solutions that are distilled from deep research on many topics. She is the author of over 50 books, with nine being Amazon best-sellers, on topics such as natural health, biblical studies, devotionals, and doctrine. Dr. Jen has been a professional educator and international conference speaker since 1999. She has a desire to help educate on holistic health and wellness through natural products and lifestyle changes with the overarching goal of supporting women in their spiritual health with Jesus.

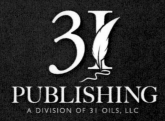

31 PUBLISHING
A DIVISION OF 31 OILS, LLC

ISBN: 979-8-32956-473-0

9 798329 564730

www.PATCHEDU.com

Made in United States
Orlando, FL
08 December 2024